Practitioner's Laboratory

By Richard T. Goldston, DVM, MS, Dip. ACVIM, Dip. ABVP
Richard D. Wilkes, DVM and
Irene M. Seybold, CVT

VETERINARY MEDICINE PUBLISHING CO.,
690 South 4th Street,
Edwardsville, Ks 66111

ISBN 0-935078-27-4

Library of Congress Catalog No. 83-051492

DEDICATION

To all practicing veterinarians who strive to continually improve their diagnostic skills and patient management methods through an increased use of the clinical pathology laboratory.

To all veterinary laboratory technicians who dedicate their time, skills and knowledge in striving for accurate laboratory results to improve animal health care.

Richard T. Goldston, DVM, MS, Dip. ACVIM, Dip. ABVP
Richard D. Wilkes, DVM
Irene M. Seybold, CVT

ACKNOWLEDGMENTS

We are very grateful for the expert help received from Veterinary Medicine Publishing Company, particularly from Sue Weller and Ray Ottinger for initiating interest in producing this publication and Dr. David Chubb, Sandra Grey, and especially Pamela Landon for expert guidance in its preparation.

CONTENTS

Reprinted from VM/SAC

PREFACE & FOREWORD

Effective treatment and control of medical disorders of companion animals can only be successful when the diagnosis of the disorder is correct. Because veterinary patients cannot verbalize their aches, pains and discomforts, greater emphasis must be put on the physical examination and history to localize the disorder to an organ system. Selective clinical laboratory tests, properly performed and interpreted can then further define the disorder and in many cases establish a specific diagnosis. It has been said that "one who depends entirely on the laboratory to make his diagnosis is probably inexperienced; one who says that he does not need a laboratory is uninformed. In either instance the patient is in danger."[1]

PRACTITIONER'S LABORATORY is an attempt to simplfy the complex subject of clinical pathology. The material is directed to the practicing veterinarian and the veterinary laboratory technician. Methodologies of performing individual tests are summarized in tables whenever possible. Simplified and concise interpretations of results and normal value ranges are given. Charts, figures, color photographs and photomicrographs and a glossary of terms are provided. Specific medical disorders of each system and their medical management are discussed when applicable.

1. Wells, B.B.: Halsten, J.A.: Clinical Pathology, 4th ed. W.B. Saunders Co., Philadelphia, Pa., 1967: p 1.

Equipment and collection techniques 1

CHAPTER 1

Selection of equipment

THE ADVANCES in veterinary medicine throughout history have continually stimulated veterinary practitioners to deliver service of higher quality to their clientele. With these advances, the clinical pathology laboratory has become an indispensable aid to veterinary practitioners in the achievement of an accurate diagnosis, valid prognosis, and proper therapy. In addition to this increase in the quality of services, the amount of work performed by a hospital can be increased by 15 to 20% with proper use of a clinical laboratory.[1]

The practitioner recognizes the large investment required to establish a practice; the return on that investment depends upon his or her ability to use profitably such ancillary aids as clinical pathology, radiology, etc. The primary goal for the clinical pathology laboratory is to make reliably available, necessary test procedures at a reasonable cost and with a fair return on the practitioner's investment. Practitioners who plan properly and who make optimal use of manpower and equipment will achieve this goal.

Essentially every veterinary hospital should have a basic clinical pathology laboratory. This basic facility should provide competency in routine hematology, urinalysis, parasitology, and blood glucose and blood urea nitrogen (BUN) measurements. Thus, the practitioner has the capability to screen patients with undiagnosed illnesses and to evaluate the response to therapy by hospitalized patients and out-patients.

Practitioners considering installing a clinical pathology laboratory should first evaluate their individual requirements in clinical pathology and the cost:benefit ratio of an in-hospital laboratory versus the use of commercial laboratories. Economics, convenience, and the practitioner's interests are all important considerations in determining the extent to which the laboratory should be developed.

The in-hospital laboratory offers convenience, and with continual use it can become very reliable. The cost advantages of an in-hospital laboratory compared to using a commercial laboratory can only be calculated by individual practitioners on the basis of conditions in their own areas. Commercial laboratory fees must be compared to the practitioner's initial investment in equipment, supplies, and hospital overhead. At times, the practitioner's needs can be met only by an in-hospital laboratory whether it be because of after-hours calls or a frequent need for special procedures the commercial laboratory does not perform.

If no commercial laboratory exists in the practice area, or if the practitioner's interests lie in clinical pathology, the in-hospital laboratory assumes much greater importance. The capability to render a quick definitive diagnosis, gained by having the laboratory in the hospital, increases clients' confidence in the veterinarian and reduces the extra visits required when samples must be sent to commercial laboratories. This in turn enhances the practitioner's own confidence.

In some instances a commercial laboratory offers more advantages than does an in-hospital laboratory. This is the situation when the practitioner lacks interest in laboratory functions or has not the time required to establish and maintain the laboratory, when the practice has a low volume of work, or when the cost of maintaining the laboratory would exceed the return on the practitioner's investment. In general, the cost is unfavorable for maintaining the capability to perform any test required less than once a week.[2]

The use of a commercial laboratory must also be considered advantageous in many instances because of the laboratory's advanced capabilities and reliability. The large volume processed by a commercial laboratory usually means more qualified personnel familiar with the latest techniques. However, if the cost of outside laboratory services is incompatible with the economic condition of the practice or if the commercial laboratory is inaccessible or is unreliable in handling veterinary specimens, then the in-hospital laboratory becomes the obvious choice.

The information presented here is offered as a guide to help the practitioner set up a new clinical pathology laboratory or improve an existing one. Advance planning is most important in establishing a laboratory. The scope of the laboratory should be limited to those tests that can be performed accurately at a cost competitive with that charged by any available commercial laboratory. Several factors influence the decision regarding which tests to be performed in the hospital laboratory. Of these factors, the most important is the volume of a test required by the hospital. Unless performed routinely, a test is not likely to be done with accuracy and precision, and the reagents are apt to become outdated and unstable. Equipment and personnel are additional factors that influence the success or failure of an in-hospital laboratory. Results of a test cannot be accurate unless the test is done on quality, calibrated equipment by a reliable technician.

The most organized system for fulfilling the needs of the practice is the panel. This approach, which employs a predetermined test schedule (screening versus specific tests) is applicable to most in-hospital laboratories. By this means a broad variety of abnormalities can be identified or ruled out of the differential diagnoses. The screening panel is a group of nonspecific tests that gives the practitioner an overview of the patient.

The panel is usually, but not always, limited to a complete blood count (CBC), urinalysis, fecal examination, and determination of blood urea nitrogen (BUN). In geographic areas where incidence of specific diseases is high (*e.g.* dirofilariasis) specific tests for these diseases may be incorporated in the routine screening profiles. Results of this panel of tests may pinpoint a diseased organ, thus indicating a need for other, more specific tests.

To have the above-mentioned capabilities, the basic laboratory should provide routine hematology, urinalysis, parasitology, and measurement of limited blood chemistries. Seventy-five percent of the work required in an in-hospital laboratory can most often be covered by this basic schedule.[3]

Equipment and supplies

When equipment is purchased, quality—not quantity—should be the main consideration. Expensive equipment, however, is no substitute for knowledge and can only be used properly by trained personnel. The volume of tests to be performed; the simplicity, reliability, versatility, and ease of operation; and availability of maintenance should all be considered when equipment is being selected.

Microscope

The microscope is the cornerstone of a well-equipped laboratory. This is one area in which the laboratory must not be compromised. Only a microscope of excellent quality should be used, since routine hematology and urinalysis cannot be performed reliably with a microscope of poor quality. When a microscope of high quality is available, procedures can easily be expanded to include semen evaluation, exfoliative cytology, and special parasitology (*i.e.* blood parasites).

The microscope in the clinical laboratory should be binocular with wide-field oculars and have a mechanical stage, flat-field objectives (10 ×, 40 ×, 100 ×), oil immersion, and a variable light source.

Centrifuges

Centrifuges are also essential to the clinical laboratory. A separate standard centrifuge and a microhematocrit centrifuge are recommended. The microhematocrit centrifuge produces the packed cell volume (PCV) which can often eliminate the need to count red blood cells and determine hemoglobin levels. For maximum packing of cells, the microhematocrit tubes should spin at 10,000 G for five minutes.

The standard centrifuge with 15-ml heads to hold test tubes is adequate for most hospital laboratories. The floating heads help to keep sediment, cells, etc. directly in the bottom of the tube, although this is seldom required. The centrifuge is used to separate serum, sediment urine, and concentrate microfilariae in heartworm tests.

Cell tabulator

A cell tabulator should also be considered essential. Although this instrument is fairly expensive in light of its limitations, it provides the only means by which cells in a blood smear can be counted accurately. The conventional cell tabulator has separate counters for each type of white blood cell. A bell rings when 100 cells have been counted.

Refractometer

A refractometer is used frequently in the clinical laboratory. Specific gravity of urine and other fluids is an important diagnostic indicator. Other values frequently determined using a refractometer include plasma proteins and total solids of body fluids. Additional advantages of the refractometer are the small amount of urine or plasma needed, plus easy and quick readings. Direct-reading scales are usually best.

The American-made instruments (American Optical TS Meter) cost from three to four times more than those made in Japan; however, the more expensive models are recommended because of their longer life expectancy and greater accuracy.

Hemocytometer

Although many hospitals are now equipped with an automated cell counter, the hemocytometer remains the basic cell-counting instrument. After the technique of using the hemocytometer has been mastered, and with the use of commercially prepared, prediluted pipettes (Unopette® — Becton-Dickinson), the hemocytometer is adequate for counting white blood cells in the clinical laboratory. This device is generally considered inaccurate for counting erythrocytes.

Colorimeters

Colorimeters are available in many sizes and price ranges. A laboratory should be equipped to determine, colorimetrically, at least blood glucose and BUN levels. Other tests can easily be added after the basic colorimeter has been purchased.

In general, results achieved with colorimeters are reasonably accurate and reproducible. This is especially true when the colorimeter is used by a reliable technician after performing the common laboratory procedures of standardizing individual tests and frequently cross-checking results against control serum.

Stains

No laboratory can be considered adequate without at least the common stains. Daily use of stains is important to minimize staining errors. There is no foolproof procedure. The most common staining problems result from using reagents of poor quality and from the technician's inattention to detail.

Although several stains are available for the many different situations a practitioner encounters, only two are required. A type of Romanovsky's stain, such as Wright's stain, is the standard to be used. The second stain should be a supravital stain, such as new methylene blue. New methylene blue is a simple and quick stain that stains only nuclear material, reticulocytes, and Heinz bodies. It is used routinely to stain blood smears from anemic animals for estimating the reticulocyte count, and also to stain urine sediment.

The "quick" stains generally do not give consistent results and thus are not routinely recommended.

Certain special stains, such as Giemsa stain for blood parasites and Shorr's stain for viral inclusion bodies, may be used but they are not essential. Because the amount of time a practitioner can spend in the laboratory is limited, he or she should become knowledgeable about only the more common stains. Some practitioners may also feel a need for Gram's stain and a fungal stain for performing microbial studies.

Laboratory log

A laboratory log should be maintained on a daily basis. The Clinical Pathology Laboratory Log published by the American Animal Hospital Association is excellent. It provides for a separate permanent record of laboratory tests performed, can be used for quick medical references, and is a source for determining frequency of individual tests performed and cost:benefit analysis of the clinical laboratory.

The instruments and equipment we have cited here are considered basic components of the veterinarian's in-hospital laboratory. Few additional expensive items would be needed in most hospitals. Certain smaller items of supplies must also be considered: microscope slides, coverslips, hematocrit tubes, blood tubes, test tubes, staining tray, timers, urine and blood chemistry assay strips, pipettes, beakers, flasks, and culture media.

REFERENCES

1. Mia, A.S.; Tierney, M.T.: Clinical Laboratory Management in Veterinary Hospitals. *Practicing Vet.* *50*(1):3; Summer, 1979.
2. Tasker, J.B.: The Veterinary Hospital Laboratory. In *The Veterinary Clinics of North America* 6(4):524; Nov. 1976.

CHAPTER 2

Colorimeters and spectrophotometers

SPECTROPHOTOMETERS and colorimeters differ primarily in the way they separate the electromagnetic light spectrum into different wave lengths. Spectrophotometers use prisms to separate the visible portion of the electromagnetic spectrum of light into wave lengths from about 300 to 1000 nanometers. Colorimeters use color filters to separate the electromagnetic spectrum of light into a few, selected wave lengths. As the number of wave lengths of light increase, so do the number and accuracy of the clinical laboratory procedures that can be performed.

Spectrophotometers and colorimeters have several basic components:

1. A power supply to furnish properly regulated electricity.
2. A device (prism or color filter) for separating the desired wave lengths of light.
3. A photocell to detect the amount of light transmitted through the specimen and to convert this light to measurable electrical energy.
4. A readout meter to display the measured electrical energy in recognizable units.

Colorimeters

Several small colorimeters have been developed for use in the in-hospital laboratory. More than 20 tests can easily be performed with these instruments. Pre-packaged, disposable reagent kits, which require no special glassware, can be used.

Most colorimeters have built-in incubators calibrated at 37 C and 100 C. Advantages and disadvantages of these instruments are summarized in Table 1. The most commonly used colorimeters are the Accu Stat® (Clay-Adams), Serometer® (Mallinckrodt), and Unimeter® (Bio-Dynamics).

TABLE 1—Advantages and Disadvantages of Small Colorimeters

Advantages	Disadvantages
1. Easy to use.	1. Costs per individual test are higher.
2. Relatively accurate.	2. Limited number of tests available.
3. No additional glassware or instruments required.	3. Reagent kits are sometimes hard to purchase.
4. Take less of the technician's time.	4. Reagent kits may have a relatively short shelf life.

TABLE 2—Advantages and Disadvantages of Small Spectrophotometers

Advantages	Disadvantages
1. Many tests can be performed.	1. Additional glassware and instruments (incubators, etc.) are required.
2. Reagent costs less per test	2. More of technician's time is needed to prepare reagents; clean glassware.
3. Reagents in bulk have a longer shelf life.	3. More technical knowledge and skill are needed to perform the tests.

Spectrophotometers

Small spectrophotometers have also been developed for use in the in-hospital laboratory. Virtually all clinical chemistry procedures can be done with these instruments. However, more time and technical knowledge is needed to perform the tests than is needed for tests with colorimeters. Prepackaged, disposable kits are also available for common chemistry procedures. But for most tests, the technician must prepare the specific amount of reagent needed from a larger supply of bulk reagents. Thus, additional glassware must be purchased and maintained.

Spectrophotometers do not have built-in incubator systems. Therefore, water baths and/or heat blocks must be purchased and maintained. Advantages and disadvantages of spectrophotometers are summarized in Table 2.

Setting standards

Standardization and quality control should be rigidly held criteria when chemistry determinations are made in the laboratory. Instruments should be standardized before each test procedure. This is done with an artificial standard of solution that gives an established value for light absorbency for each test procedure. Before a test is performed on the unknown or test serum sample, the artificial standard is tested. The instrument is then calibrated to the proper level of absorbency.

Measurements of quality control are taken from control serum samples that have been statistically analyzed and contain a known amount of a compound. The entire laboratory procedure is performed on the sample. Results should be close to the known value of the control sample. Control sera with values in both normal and abnormal ranges for each test can be purchased from American Scientific Products, Inc.

CHAPTER 3

Collection and preservation of specimens

THE HANDLING OF SPECIMENS for the laboratory is not usually given its due importance. One must consider as separate links in a chain of events, each step from collection and preservation of the specimen to the final performance and interpretation of the laboratory test. Improper technique anywhere along that chain of events will adversely affect the results of the procedure.

Blood

Blood is probably the most common specimen collected for the clinical pathology laboratory. Although not often considered when a blood sample is taken, body physiology is altered by many external stimuli, such as excitement, fear, and even physical exercise. Optimally, blood samples should be taken after the animal has been fasted for 12 hours, and without inducing undue excitement or fear. Usually 10 ml of blood is adequate for most chemistry panels.

The blood sample should be placed in a sterile container with proper anticoagulant, if needed. Tubes of up to 15-ml capacity, with or without anticoagulant, are commercially available (Vacutainer® —Becton-Dickinson) and are very convenient.

Each of the blood's many constituents should be protected from detrimental conditions. Careful mixing is necessary when anticoagulants are used. When possible, blood smears should be prepared immediately as the specimen is withdrawn from the animal, without using anticoagulants. Improper use of anticoagulants can interfere with staining and can significantly decrease the PCV by crenation of erythrocytes.

Hemolysis is another common cause of inaccurate test results. Frequent causes of hemolysis are rough handling of the specimen, moisture, osmotic imbalances, excessive vacuum, forcibly expelling blood through the needle, chemical contamination, and freezing and thawing.

Venous samples are most often used because they are easy to collect, but arterial blood is occasionally required for measuring such factors as arterial blood gases. Properly cleaned areas rich in capillary beds (*i.e.* ear, toenails, etc.) are acceptable for collection of blood from puppies and kittens when necessary.

In processing blood specimens, one must know whether plasma, serum, or whole blood is required for the test to be performed. When these specimens are collected, processing should begin as soon as possible, preferably within one-half hour. Whole blood should be stored under refrigeration, *not frozen*. Serum is the noncellular portion of clotted blood, and plasma is the noncellular portion of anticoagulated blood. Both should be pipetted from the cellular sediment immediately after centrifugation. Either plasma or serum should be frozen if testing is to be delayed more than 12 hours after collection; otherwise, refrigeration is recommended.

The following anticoagulants are used to store blood, synovial fluid, and cerebrospinal fluid.

1. Ethylenediaminetetraacetate (EDTA)

EDTA prevents coagulation by chelating calcium. It is available in both dry and liquid forms. The dry form is used at the rate of 2 mg/ml blood, the liquid form at the rate of one drop/5 ml of blood. EDTA is useful for short-term storing or shipping of blood. Refrigeration of the blood sample is always advisable if it will not be tested on the day it is collected.

EDTA is the anticoagulant of choice for preserving cells and cellular morphology. Staining progresses with little interference if EDTA is used in the proper concentration. When excess EDTA is used the PCV will decrease significantly due to erythrocyte crenation. Automated cell counters work well with blood to which EDTA has been added.

2. Heparin

Heparin is relatively expensive, but only very small quantities are used. Heparin prevents coagulation by interfering with the conversion of prothrombin to thrombin. By coating the inside of the syringe with heparin, enough of the anticoagulant is usually provided to prevent coagulation of the sample.

Heparin is useful for immediate transfusions and routine hematology procedures. It prevents coagulation for 10 to 12 hours. One disadvantage is its adverse effects on the stainability of leukocytes.

3. Oxylates

Oxylates combine with calcium to prevent coagulation. They are inexpensive and cause little distortion of cells within one hour. The ammonium oxylates cannot be used for measuring BUN. Ammonium oxylates increase the size of erythrocytes, whereas potassium oxylates reduce the size of erythrocytes, thus influencing the PCV.

4. Fluorides

Sodium and potassium fluoride are used primarily to preserve glucose. The required concentration is 10mg fluoride/100 ml blood. This process is unnecessary if the determination is performed immediately after the blood sample is withdrawn. Fluoride also inhibits enzymes. For this reason it cannot be used to determine serum glutamic-pyruvic transaminase (SGPT), serum glutamic-oxaloacetic transaminase (SGOT), or lipase levels.

5. Sodium Citrate

Sodium citrate is used routinely in blood stored for transfusion. It is not recommended for hematology or determination of blood chemistry.

Urine

Results of urinalysis can reveal many metabolic problems in addition to certain diseases of kidneys, urinary bladder, and liver. Because urine is an excellent bacterial culture medium, bacterial overgrowth can cause alterations in urinary constituents.[1]

The optimal specimen is 15 ml, examined immediately. As urine ages after collection, urea-splitting bacteria increase the urine pH, causing autolyzation of cells and dissolution of casts. Of the 15 ml, 10 ml should be centrifuged and the supernatant poured off, leaving 0.5 ml of sediment for the microscopic examination. This allows for some degree of standardization which permits the technician, with practice, to interpret more accurately the various degrees of abnormalities.

Urine can be collected in several ways: by catheterization, by cystocentesis, by manual expression, or by catching a voided specimen. The best routine is to collect in an uncontaminated container, an early-morning, voided midstream sample. Specimens for culture should be collected by cystocentesis using a 20- to 24-gauge, 1½- to 2-inch needle. Cystocentesis should not be attempted if the bladder cannot be palpated. For quantitative analysis, a 24-hour total output is required.

Refrigeration is recommended if the urine sample cannot be examined immediately. When the sample is to be examined after refrigeration, it should be first allowed to warm to room temperature.

Toluene is a good preservative for urine. Just a layer of toluene over the urine serves the purpose. Formalin alters the chemical constituents in urine, but is good for preserving urine sediment and cell structure. It is used at the rate of five to 10 drops of a 10% solution to 10 ml of urine. Sodium fluoride can be used in urine to inhibit glycolysis and bacterial growth.

Other common specimens

For the most valid results, cerebrospinal fluid should be taken aseptically and examined within 30 minutes. The collection site is the cisterna magna. The cerebrospinal fluid should be free of blood and contaminants.

Histologic sections are prepared by forming 1/4- to 3/8-inch sections of normal and abnormal tissue. Formalin 10% is used as a preservative at a ratio of 10 parts formalin:1 part tissue. Formaldehyde (40%) is mixed at a ratio of 1:9 with water to form 10% formalin. The formalin can be buffered by adding 4.0 gm monobasic sodium phosphate and 6.5 gm dibasic sodium phosphate to 1000 ml of 10% formalin.

When an animal is suspected of having rabies, the intact head is sent in a plastic or metal container to a state diagnostic laboratory or county health department. The head of a rabies suspect may not be mailed. Railway, air express, and bus are common means of transportation. The outside of the package should specify "Animal Species" and "Call on Arrival". Refrigeration—*not freezing*—is usually recommended.

Materials used for toxicology include necropsy specimens, tissues, blood, excretory products, feeds, water, and plants. Liberal amounts should be collected from several locations and placed in separate clean plastic bags. All specimens should be refrigerated. When poisoning is suspected, the stomach contents, blood, urine, kidney, and liver tissue usually suffice for laboratory analysis.

When requested to do so, microbiologic laboratories supply information on the collection and preservation of specimens usually submitted. Sterile tubes and containers for most microbiologic specimens are commercially available. Samples should be collected before therapy is instituted. Viral samples must be frozen and shipped in tightly sealed containers. Skin scrapings and fungal cultures may be shipped in sterile culture tubes. Milk samples are usually collected for a variety of tests. These samples should be collected aseptically; they may

Guidelines for Collecting and Preserving the Blood Specimen

1. Collect fasting samples (lipemia interferes with many measurements).
2. Collect samples before beginning treatment (drugs may greatly alter results of laboratory tests).
3. Attempt to obtain samples from calm animals (excitement may alter several factors).
4. Jugular venipuncture is preferred (larger veins yield far more blood and are less subject to hemolysis).
5. Draw enough blood to perform all tests. Fill each tube completely. Tests require a specified amount of blood; further dilution can cause erroneous results.
6. Place blood in proper tubes. Tubes with EDTA anticoagulant are required for hematology. Tubes without anticoagulants (serum) are required for chemistries.
7. If hematology is needed, make two good blood smears with fresh blood and submit with each request for a complete blood count. Anticoagulants can alter leukocyte morphology, making identification of leukocytes difficult.
8. For blood chemistries, submit separated serum when possible. Optimally, allow 30 minutes (never more than two hours) for the sample to clot. Centrifuge specimens at a speed of 2000 rpm to 3000 rpm for 10 minutes and extract serum. Separation of serum from red blood cells is mandatory if samples are to be mailed.
9. If possible, refrigerate samples until they are analyzed or picked up for delivery to the laboratory. Freeze serum or plasma samples if testing is to be delayed.[3]

be either refrigerated or frozen.

Bone marrow

Examination of bone marrow in the clinical laboratory is becoming more routine. The technique can be performed with or without the patient under general anesthesia, but local anesthetics and tranquilizers are routinely used. A sterile bone-marrow aspiration needle or a 14- to 16-gauge needle with a stylet is adequate.

The iliac crest and proximal femur are the most common sites in the dog. A 10-ml syringe is used to aspirate a couple of drops of marrow. The vacuum should be carefully controlled to minimize the possibility of rupturing bone-marrow sinusoids and diluting the sample with peripheral blood.

The sternum is a common site in cattle, horses, and sheep. The seventh rib, at a point between the upper and middle third of the rib, can also be used.

To perform bone-marrow aspiration in a cat, an intramedullary pin can be used to bore a hole in the trochanteric fossa of the femur, which is the most common route of collection in cats. Anesthesia is usually required for this procedure and smears should be made immediately after the specimen is collected. After the smear has dried, any of the common stains can be used. If an anticoagulant is needed, EDTA is recommended.

REFERENCE

1. Morgan, H.C.: Selecting Basic Laboratory Equipment. *VM/SAC* *61*(2):170-172; Feb. 1966.

CHAPTER 4

Evaluation of the erythrocytes:

hematocrit and hemoglobin determinations

Hematocrit determination

The hematocrit (HCT) is the percentage of blood comprised of red blood cells. The test is one of the easiest, most accurate, and most informative for evaluating the erythrocytes. When the HCT is determined by centrifugal methods, the product is called the packed cell volume (PCV).

In the past, the PCV was determined by the macrohematocrit centrifugation method of Wintrobe. The Wintrobe method is reasonably accurate and offers the advantage of using the same blood sample to determine the erythrocyte sedimentation rate (ESR) and to estimate the total white blood cell count. However, the Wintrobe method requires at least 1 ml of blood and 30 minutes of centrifugation. Also, the Wintrobe tubes must be cleaned before they are reused. Due to these disadvantages, the high-speed capillary-tube method (microhematocrit) has become the method preferred by most veterinary laboratories.

The microhematocrit

The microhematocrit method uses disposable capillary tubes about 0.55 mm to 1.2 mm in diameter and 75 mm long. They are filled by capillary action from a tube of unclotted blood. The capillary tubes are available either plain or heparinized and either precalibrated or noncalibrated.

When noncalibrated capillary tubes are used, a special linear chart such as Critocap Micro-Hematocrit Tube Reader (Biologic Research Inc., St. Louis, Mo.) is required to determine the PCV. After the filled capillary tube is centrifuged, it is placed over the reader card with the top of the plasma column aligned with the 100% line and the bottom of the packed red blood cells aligned with the 0% line. The line that intersects the top of the packed red blood cell column represents the PCV in percent.

When precalibrated capillary tubes are properly used in calibrated microhematocrit centrifuges, the PCV can be read directly from the calibration line on the microhematocrit centrifuge head. The microhematocrit method requires only five minutes of centrifugation and only a small amount of blood. With proper technique the method is accurate to ±0.5%.[1]

The major disadvantage to the microhematocrit method is that it requires a special centrifuge to hold the capillary tubes. However, such centrifuges have a long life expectancy, are simple to use, and can centrifuge the specimens at greater than 10,000 G. This results in complete packing of the erythrocytes in five minutes.

Electronic cell counters

Electronic devices that count particle size, such as the Coulter Counters (Coulter Electronics, Hialeah, Fla.) can also measure PCV. Measurement by these devices is also based on calculations from red blood cell counts and volume measurements. When calculated by this method, the PCV is not influenced by anticoagulant type or ratio of anticoagulant to quantity of blood.[2] There is, however, a potential for error due to the complexity of erythrocyte measurements and the fact that most of the instruments are standardized with human blood.

Interpretation of the hematocrit

Several technical factors can cause errors in measuring the PCV of domestic animals. Prolonged occlusion of the vein can cause venous stasis and increase the PCV as much as 5%. In hyperexcited animals, release of epinephrine and subsequent splenic contractions can increase the venous PCV by 10-15%, because the PCV of splenic blood is approximately 80%. Excessive use of the anticoagulant, EDTA, can reduce PCV as much as 37%.[3]

The normal PCV in the dog is 37-55% (mean 45%). The normal PCV for the cat is 24-45% (mean 37%).[4] A PCV value below the normal range for the species usually indicates anemia. Anemias will be discussed in detail in a subsequent chapter.

A PCV value above the normal range indicates polycythemia. The most common form of this condition is relative polycythemia due to dehydration or splenic contraction. Absolute polycythemia is seen most often as a secondary sequella to chronic hypoxemia, as in cardiopulmonary disease. Rarely, absolute polycythemia may be the primary polycythemia vera associated with active excess production of erythrocytes.

The PCV reflects the percentage of concentration of red blood cells in the peripheral blood. It is not a measurement of the total mass of red blood cells. The PCV may be low in hydremic conditions such as pregnancy, hypoproteinemia, iatrogenic overhydration, etc., but the total mass of red blood cells may be normal. Conversely, an animal in shock may have an elevated or normal PCV accompanied by hemoconcentration yet the total red blood cell mass may be reduced due to loss of blood. These variables must be considered when the PCV is interpreted.

Microhematocrit centrifugation can be used to measure PCV simply and accurately, and simultaneously to acquire other useful information. The plasma layer above the packed cell column can be observed for color and transparency. Normal plasma in dogs and cats is colorless and nonturbid. In icterus, plasma is yellow and nonturbid. In hyperlipidemic conditions the plasma is white and turbid. In hemoglobinemia, plasma is red and nonturbid.

After the plasma column has been observed for color and transparency, it can be examined microscopically for microfilariae. If present, microfilariae are usually undulating at the point where the plasma and buffy coat meet. The plasma column can also be used to determine the total plasma protein level by refractometry, and the fibrinogen concentration by heat precipitation and refractometry.

When used to its fullest extent, a simply performed PCV can indicate the presence or absence of anemia, polycythemia, icterus, lipemia, and hemoglobinemia. With little added effort the total plasma protein and fibrinogen levels can be determined and a screen test for microfilariae performed.

Hemoglobin determination

Hemoglobin (Hb), the main component of the erythrocyte, is a conjugated protein that serves as the vehicle to transport oxygen and carbon dioxide. When fully saturated, each gram of hemoglobin carries approximately 1.36 ml of oxygen.[1] The total red cell mass of a normal dog weighing 44 lb (20 kg) should, therefore, be capable of carrying approximately 250 ml of oxygen.

Hemoglobin determination is not as frequently performed in veterinary medicine as is the PCV. Alone, it provides no clinical advantage over the PCV. However, the hemoglobin determination combined with the PCV can give a reliable index of hemoglobin concentration in the red blood cells.

Hemoglobin can be measured as oxyhemoglobin or converted to one of its derivatives as acid hematin, alkaline hematin, or cyanmethemoglobin. The measurement can be made visually by color-comparison charts, or photoelectrically with a colorimeter. The colorimetric measurement of cyanmethemoglobin is the most accurate and most often used method in veterinary clinical pathology.

Hemoglobin concentration is measured in grams per deciliter (g/dl). It is the most direct indication of the capacity of the blood to transport oxygen. If the erythrocytes are of normal size, as determined by examination of the blood smear, the hemoglobin concentration should be approximately one-third of the PCV or, expressed mathematically:

$$\frac{PCV}{3} = \text{Hb in g/dl.}$$

Interpretation of hemoglobin value

The normal hemoglobin concentration for the dog ranges from 12 to 18 g/dl (mean 15 g/dl). The normal hemoglobin concentration for the cat ranges from 8 to 15 g/dl (mean 12 g/dl). Interpretation of hemoglobin values parallels that of the PCV values; that is, values below the normal range indicate anemia, and values above the normal range indicate polycythemia—most commonly hemoconcentration due to dehydration.

When combined with the PCV, the mean corpuscular hemoglobin concentration (MCHC) can be mathematically calculated by the formula:

$$\frac{\text{Hb X 100}}{PCV} = \text{MCHC g/dl.}$$

This gives an index of the percent hemoglobin concentration in the red blood cells. The normal MCHC for the dog is 32 to 36 g/dl. For the cat, the normal MCHC is 30 to 36 g/dl.[4] Values below the normal range are seen in animals with iron deficiency anemias and any condition inducing reticulocytosis, *i.e.* regenerative anemias. Values above the normal range are usually associated with *in vivo* or *in vitro* hemolysis.

Reduced hemoglobin is hemoglobin in which the iron is unassociated with the oxygen molecule and the heme component is reversibly combined with carbon dioxide. When the heme molecules are associated with oxygen, the hemoglobin is referred to as *oxyhemoglobin*.

In both reduced hemoglobin and oxyhemoglobin, the iron is in the ferrous state. When iron is oxidized to the ferric state, methemoglobin is formed and the molecule loses its capacity to carry oxygen or carbon dioxide. Thus the molecule becomes an "inactive" hemoglobin. Abnormal amounts of methemoglobin result in functional anemia with cyanosis. Specific examples of methemoglobinemic conditions in domestic animals include nitrate toxicities in all species and acetaminophen (Tylenol® — McNeil) toxicity in feline species.

Cyanosis occurs when the reduced hemoglobin level exceeds 5 g/dl. In extremely anemic animals with total hemoglobin levels less than 5 g/dl, the oxygen-carrying capacity of the blood will be significantly impaired, but cyanosis cannot be detected clinically.

REFERENCES

1. Ettinger, S.J.: *Textbook of Veterinary Internal Medicine*, Vol. 2. W.B. Saunders Co., Philadelphia, Pa., 1975.
2. Davidsohn, I.; Henry, J.B.: *Clinical Diagnosis by Laboratory Methods*, 15th ed. W.B. Saunders Co., Philadelphia, Pa., 1974.
3. Penny, R.H. *et al*: Some Observations on the Effect of the Concentration of Ethylenediamine Tetraacetic Acid (EDTA) on the Packed Cell Volume of Domesticated Animals. *Br. Vet. J. 126*:383; 1970a.
4. Schalm, O.W. *et al: Veterinary Hematology*, 3rd ed. Lea & Febiger, Philadelphia, Pa., 1975.

CHAPTER 5

Evaluation of the erythrocytes:

total erythrocyte count, erythrocyte indices and sedimentation rate

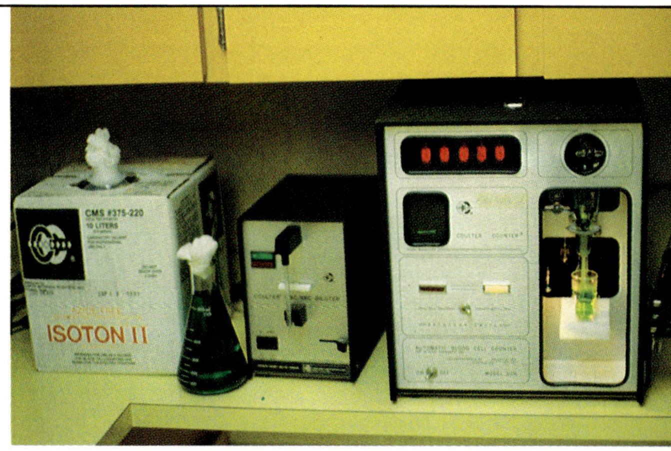

Figure 1—The Coulter Counter Model D2N.

Blood-cell counting

Quantitative measurements of any of the formed elements in the blood (*i.e.*, erythrocytes, leukocytes, and thrombocytes) are concerned with the concentration of each element in a microliter of blood. In the past, the unit of measurement for the cell counts was expressed as cubic millimeters (cumm or mm^3). However, for metric standardization, it is now recommended that all units of volume measurement be expressed in liters. Since 1 cubic millimeter (mm^3) is equal to 1.00003 microliters (μl), the microliter is now considered to be the equivalent measurement and is the preferred term.

Any cell-counting procedure involves four basic steps: 1) diluting the blood, 2) sampling the dilution into a measured volume, 3) counting the cells in that volume, and 4) converting the cell count to number of cells per microliter.

The erythrocyte count

There are two basic methods for counting erythrocytes: the hemocytometer and the electronic-particle counter. The hemocytometer is considered too inaccurate for counting erythrocytes, and its use is generally not recommended.

Advances in electronics have led to the development of many different, small, table-top electronic cell counters (*Figures 1-3*). These electronic cell counters, now available in many price ranges, have various capabilities and conveniences. The more expensive models can count erythrocytes and leukocytes, provide hemoglobin and hematocrit values, and calculate the erythrocyte indices—giving digital readouts for all values. The less expensive models perform only erythrocyte and leukocyte counts. The electronic counters are accurate, reliable, and easy to use.

Because the hemocytometer method is generally inaccurate and unreliable for counting erythrocytes, only the electronic counting methods are recommended and discussed here.

Electronic counting of erythrocytes

The electronic erythrocyte-counting methods most widely used today employ either of two principles:

1. Cells passing through an aperture cause changes in electronic resistance and are counted as voltage pulses. This principle is used in the Coulter Counters (Coulter Electronics, Hialeah, Fla.), Mallinckrodt cell

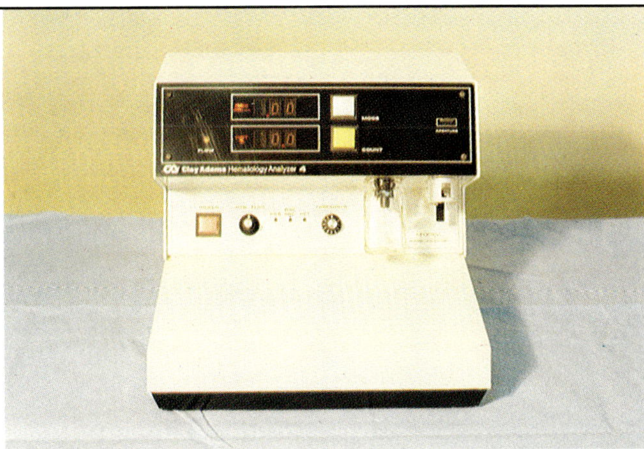

Figure 2—The Clay Adams Hematology Analyzer 4.

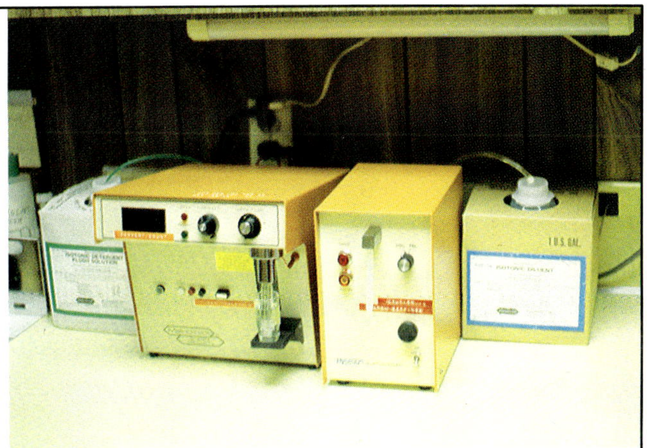

Figure 3—The Mallinckrodt Cell Counter 390.

counters (Mallinckrodt Inc., Laboratory Products Division, Bohemia, N.Y.), and Clay-Adams cell counters (Clay-Adams, Inc., Parsippany, N.J.).

2. Cells passing through a flow-cell deflect a beam of light. A photomultiplier converts this light to electronic pulses and counts them. This principle is used in the much more expensive cell counters, such as the Technicon Hemalog® (Technicon Co., Tarrytown, N.Y.) and the Hemac® (Ortho-Instrument, Division of Johnson and Johnson, Westwood, Mass.).[1]

Interpretation of total erythrocyte count

The normal range for total erythrocyte counts for the dog is $5.5 \times 10^6/\mu l$ to $8.5 \times 10^6/\mu l$ (mean $6.8 \times 10^6/\mu l$). Normal range for the cat is $5.0 \times 10^6/\mu l$ to $10.0 \times 10^6/\mu l$ (mean $7.5 \times 10^6/\mu l$).[2]

A total erythrocyte count below the normal for the species usually indicates anemia. Anemia will be discussed in detail in a subsequent section.

A total erythrocyte count above the normal range for the species indicates polycythemia. Most commonly the polycythemia is a relative polycythemia secondary to hemoconcentration resulting from dehydration or splenic contraction. Absolute polycythemia is seen most often as a secondary sequella to chronic hypoxemia, as in cardiopulmonary disease. Rarely, absolute polycythemia may be the primary polycythemia vera associated with excessive production of erythrocytes.[3]

Erythrocyte indices

The erythrocyte indices were introduced by Wintrobe to provide objective standards, rather than subjective impressions, for the study of anemias.[4] The erythrocyte indices include: mean corpuscular volume (MCV), mean corpuscular hemoglobin (MCH), and mean corpuscular hemoglobin concentration (MCHC). The basic hematologic values needed to determine the erythrocyte indices are erythrocyte count, hemoglobin, and hematocrit.

MCV

The MCV is the average volume of the individual erythrocyte. In the past, this measurement has been expressed in cubic microns (μ^3), but with metric standardization, it is now expressed in femtoliters (fl). One femtoliter equals 10^{-15} liters, which equals one cubic micron. The MCV is calculated from the formula:

$$MCV = \frac{\text{Hematocrit} \times 10}{\text{Erythrocyte count}}$$

The normal MCV range for the dog is 60 to 77 fl (mean 70 fl). The normal range for the cat is 39 to 55 fl (mean 45 fl).

Values below the normal range for the species indicate microcytosis (microcytic anemia). Microcytosis usually is due to defective maturation of cytoplasm. Some nutritional factors (*e.g.*, iron deficiency) can cause extra cell divisions in the bone marrow, resulting in smaller erythrocytes.

Values above the normal range for the species indicate macrocytosis. The most common cause of erythrocyte macrocytosis in the dog and cat is normal response to anemia; *i.e.* reticulocytosis. Erythrocytic macrocytosis not associated with responsive anemia (reticulocytosis) reflects defects of maturation in the nucleus. These changes are seen in some cases of vitamin deficiency (folic acid, vitamin B_{12}), some forms of liver disease, and some myeloproliferative diseases.

MCH

The MCH is the hemoglobin content of the average individual erythrocyte. It is a weight measurement formerly expressed as micromicrogram ($\mu\mu g$), but with metric standardization the preferred unit is now the picogram (pg). The MCH is calculated from the formula:

$$MCH = \frac{\text{Hemoglobin} \times 10}{\text{Erythrocyte count}}$$

The normal range of MCH for the dog is 19.5 to 24.5 pg (mean 22.8 pg). The normal range for the cat is 12.5 to 17.5 pg (mean 15.5 pg).

Values below the normal range are associated with microcytic anemia. Values above the normal range can be associated with macrocytic anemias. The MCH will be erroneously elevated in *in vivo* or *in vitro* hemolysis because the extracellular hemoglobin is measured. The survival time of macrocytic erythrocytes produced in response to marked erythropoietin stimulation is less than one-half that of normal erythrocytes. This accelerated destruction of erythrocytes is probably related to glucose deprivation in tissues when macrocytes become sequestrated due to their large size.[5]

TABLE 1—Factors That May Influence Erythrocyte Sedimentation Rate*

Increase Rate	Decrease Rate
1. Increased rouleau	1. Decreased rouleau
2. Increased fibrinogen	2. Increased albumin
3. Decreased albumin	3. Hemoconcentration
4. Increased globulin	4. Low ambient temperature
5. Increased cholesterol	5. Decreased plasma specific gravity
6. Decreased hematocrit	6. Delay before testing
7. X-ray irradiation	7. Short tube
8. Pregnancy (dog)	8. Decreased tube diameter
9. High room temperature	9. Excess anticoagulant
10. Increased plasma specific gravity	10. Sulfonamides
11. Excessive angle to tube	11. Glucocorticoids
12. Long tube	12. ACTH
13. Leukocytosis	13. Poikilocytosis-anisocytosis
14. Chronic interstitial nephritis	

* Reprinted in part from Morgan, H.C.: *Practitioner's Laboratory.* Veterinary Medicine Publishing Co., Inc., Bonner Springs, Kans., 1971.

TABLE 2—Relative Anticipated Erythrocyte Sedimentation Rate (in mm) of Canine Blood in One Hour for PCV Values from 10% to 48%.*

PCV	ESR	PCV	ESR	PCV	ESR
10	79	23	40	36	14
11	76	24	38	37	13
12	73	25	36	38	12
13	70	26	34	39	11
14	67	27	32	40	10
15	64	28	30	41	9
16	61	29	28	42	8
17	58	30	26	43	7
18	55	31	24	44	6
19	52	32	22	45	5
20	49	33	20	46	4
21	46	34	18	47	3
22	43	35	16	48	2

* Reprinted in part from Schalm, O.W. *et al: Veterinary Hematology,* 3rd ed. Lea & Febiger, Philadelphia, Pa., 1975.

MCHC

The MCHC is the average hemoglobin concentration/100 ml of packed erythrocytes and is expressed in percent. The MCHC is calculated from the formula:

$$\text{MCHC} = \frac{\text{Hemoglobin} \times 100}{\text{PCV}}$$

The MCHC is the most accurate of the erythrocyte indices because it does not depend on the erythrocyte count. The MCHC range for most mammals is 32 to 36%.

Values below the normal range are seen in hypochromic anemias and/or regenerative anemias in which reticulocytes contain less than a full complement of hemoglobin.

The MCHC is greater than normal only when there is a significant number of spherocytic erythrocytes, as associated with immune-mediated anemias. The MCHC will be erroneously elevated in *in vivo* or *in vitro* hemolysis because the extracellular hemoglobin is measured.

The erythrocyte sedimentation rate (ESR)

The ESR indicates the rate of sedimentation or settling of the erythrocytes when they are collected in an anticoagulant and placed in a special tube. This value is influenced by many factors, and determination of the ESR is at best a screening test which can indicate (by increased ESR) a need for more extensive studies.

In general, the factors that significantly affect the ESR can be subdivided into plasma factors and erythrocyte factors.

Plasma factors

Elevation of some plasma proteins, especially fibrinogen and globulin, favors more rapid sedimentation of the erythrocytes. The increased fibrinogen levels cause an increase in rouleau formation (a coin-stacking, clumping phenomenon of erythrocytes). When erythrocytes clump in rouleau formation, the increased weight of the clumped cells greatly accelerates the ESR.

Other plasma factors that can accelerate the ESR are elevated plasma cholesterol, and decreased albumin levels as seen in hypoproteinemia.

Erythrocyte factors

Decreased numbers of erythrocytes accelerate the ESR by changing the erythrocyte-plasma ratio, thus increasing rouleau formation. Microcytic erythrocytes, as seen in cases of iron deficiency anemia, decrease the ESR; whereas macrocytic erythrocytes in extremely regenerative anemias with high reticulocyte counts accelerate the ESR. Table 1 includes most factors that affect the ESR.

Methods to determine ESR

Several methods and tubes are available for determining the ESR, but the method of choice uses the Wintrobe tube. The Wintrobe tube is filled to the top of the 100-mm scale with anticoagulated blood, and placed in a vertical position at room temperature. After exactly 60 minutes, the bottom of the surface meniscus to the top of the column of erythrocytes is recorded (in millimeters) as the ESR.

In order to evaluate the influence of disease alone on the ESR, the ESR must be corrected to the packed cell volume (PCV). The corrected ESR is calculated by subtracting the observed ESR from the normal sedimentation for the PCV of the patient at the time of testing. Anticipated ESR values for each PCV unit from 10% to 48% of dog blood are listed in Table 2.

REFERENCES

1. Davidsohn, I.; Henry, J.B.: *Clinical Diagnosis by Laboratory Methods*, 15th ed. W.B. Saunders Co., Philadelphia, Pa. 1974.
2. Schalm, O.W. *et al: Veterinary Hematology*, 3rd ed. Lea & Febiger, Philadelphia, Pa., 1975.
3. Goldston, R.T. *et al*: The Basic Clinical Pathology Laboratory—3: Evaluation of the Erythrocytes: Hematocrit and Hemoglobin Determinations. *VM/SAC 75*(3):407-410; 1980.
4. Wintrobe, M.M.: *Clinical Hematology.* Lea & Febiger, Philadelphia, Pa., 1967.
5. Card, R.T. *et al*: Life Span and Autohemolysis of Macrocytic Erythrocytes Produced in Response to Hemorrhage. *Am. J. Physiol. 216*:974; 1969.

CHAPTER 6

Evaluation of the blood smear

EXAMINATION of the blood smear can be one of the more informative procedures performed on a blood specimen. Unfortunately, this procedure is often relegated to a commercial laboratory, incompletely performed, or even omitted. Improper technique in preparing and staining the smears and lack of confidence in interpretation are the main reasons for incomplete use of the procedure.

The blood smear can be made on commercially available precleaned glass slides or coverslips. If possible, the blood smear should be made immediately after the specimen is collected from the patient and without the use of an anticoagulant. If the blood specimen has been collected and preserved in an anticoagulant, the sample should be gently mixed before the smear is prepared.

Preparation of the slide

There are two basic techniques for preparing blood smears: the glass-slide method and the glass-coverslip method.[1]

The glass-slide method

This method is the most widely used because preparation and handling of the smear are easy. Also, more students are taught this method because schools use automated blood-staining equipment that can be used only with the glass-slide method.

To prepare the glass-slide smear, a clean, dust-free slide is laid on a flat surface. A small drop of blood is placed about 1 cm from the end of the slide. A second slide (the spreader slide) is placed in front of the drop of blood at a 30° to 40° angle and drawn back until it touches the drop. The blood will spread out along the touching end of the spreader slide. The spreader slide is then quickly and smoothly pushed forward. The smear should be rapidly dried by waving, fanning, or blowing.

If the procedure has been performed correctly, the blood smear has a smooth, even appearance and is free of ridges, waves, and holes. If the drop of blood was adequate, the thin, feathered edge of the blood smear should be about 2 cm long.

The main disadvantage of the glass-slide method is that the blood smears are usually thicker, making drying slower and causing contraction artifacts of the cells and unequal distribution of leukocytes. The unequal distribution of leukocytes

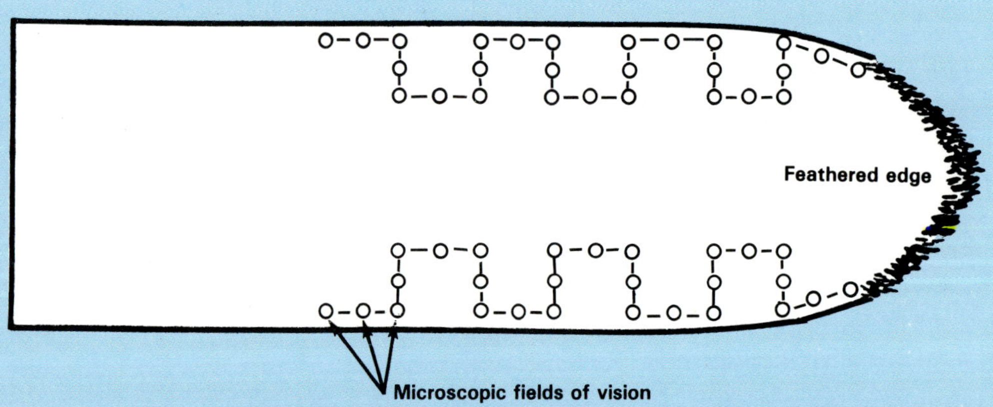

Figure 1
Performing the differential blood count by use of the battlement method.

TABLE 1—Preparation of Wright's Stain

Materials

1. Wright's Stain Crystalline—25 g (Harleco #376-25) or Wright's Blood Stain—10 packets of 0.5-g each (Harleco #508).
2. Methyl Alcohol—anhydrous, absolute, methanol acetone-free (Mallinckrodt #3016).

Preparation

0.5 g powder/300 ml absolute methyl alcohol.

Place 0.5 g powder in a mortar and slowly add 300 ml of methyl alcohol to the dye, grinding the mixture and pouring the supernate into a dry dark bottle. Continue adding methyl alcohol to the powder in the mortar, grinding and pouring until all 300 ml of methyl alcohol is used. Do not allow the mixture to contact water or other chemicals. Age the stain. The longer the stain is aged, the better its quality. Filter small quantities of the stain from the stock solution for use.

is manifest by a tendency of the neutrophils and monocytes to accumulate at the margins of the smear and the lymphocytes to accumulate centrally.

Because the leukocytes are distributed unequally, the battlement method (*Figure 1*) is used to perform the differential count of white blood cells.[2] This method involves counting the leukocytes in three horizontal fields at the edge of the smear, followed by two vertical fields toward the center of the smear, followed by two more horizontal fields, and then two fields vertically back toward the edge of the smear. This procedure is followed until 200 leukocytes are counted and differentiated.

The glass-coverslip method

This method is widely recommended and is our preference. It is the least used because considerable practice is needed to obtain good results.

The coverslips used should be new 22 × 22, No. 1 or No. 1½ thickness. Number 2 coverslips are too thick for use with oil immersion. Before they are used, the coverslips should be cleaned with alcohol and dried with lint-free tissue.

While a coverslip is held by its edge, a small drop of blood is deposited on its center. This can be done by blowing a small amount of blood from a microhematocrit tube. Another coverslip is laid diagonally over the first in such a way that the two coverslips form an eight-point star. The blood should spread evenly and quickly in a "sunburst" pattern between the two surfaces. Just as the blood stops spreading, the coverslips are pulled quickly apart on a plane parallel to their surfaces, not by lifting. The blood smear should be rapidly dried by waving, fanning, or blowing.

The advantages of the coverslip method are that the blood smear is thin and dries fast and that cells are left with fewer contraction artifacts and distributed equally. With equal distribution of the leukocytes, no special procedures are needed for performing the differential count.

The disadvantages of the coverslip method are that more practice is needed to become proficient in making coverslip smears and that coverslip smears must be mounted on a glass slide after they have been stained and before they can be examined microscopically. These are minor problems, considering the improved quality of the blood smear obtained by this method.

Staining

Ideally, the blood smear should be stained as soon as possible after it has dried. If a few hours will lapse before the blood smear is to be stained, it can be chemically fixed by immersion in absolute methyl alcohol for one minute and allowed to air-dry. If blood smears are left unfixed or unstained, the dried plasma stains and produces a precipitous hazy-blue background. Proper chemical fixation stabilizes the cells and prevents continual cellular degeneration.

Although several stains are available for the many situations a practitioner encounters, only two are required. A type of Romanowsky stain, such as Wright's stain, is the standard. The second stain should be supravital, such as new methylene blue. By becoming fully acquainted with the characteristics of these stains and the methods for using them, one can obtain consistently good results.[3]

Wright's stain can be purchased premixed or can be prepared in the laboratory by using Wright's powder and absolute methyl alcohol. The best and most consistent results can be obtained by using stain from a large quantity prepared from commercial Wright's powder (*Table 1*). The longer the

Figure 2—Feline erythrocytes with Hemobartonella organisms.

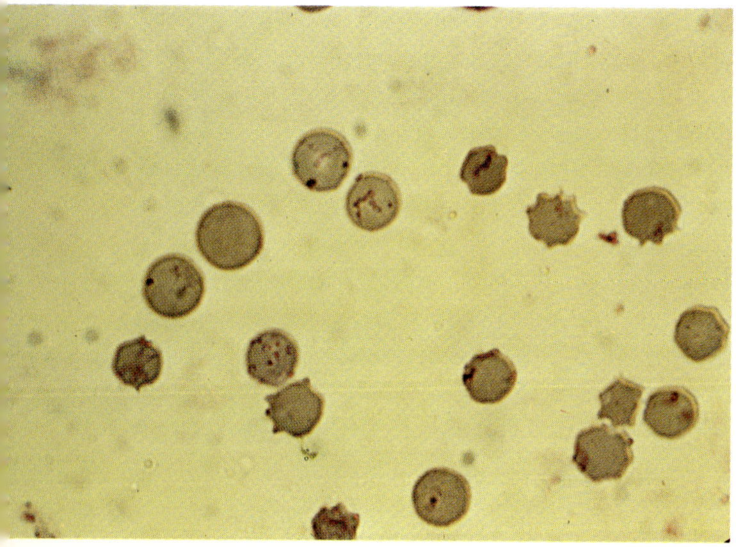

Figure 3—Equine erythrocytes with Babesia organisms.

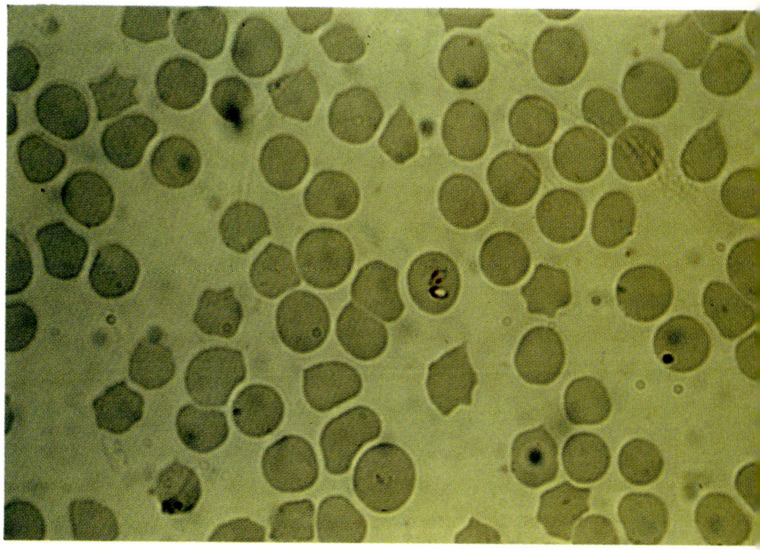

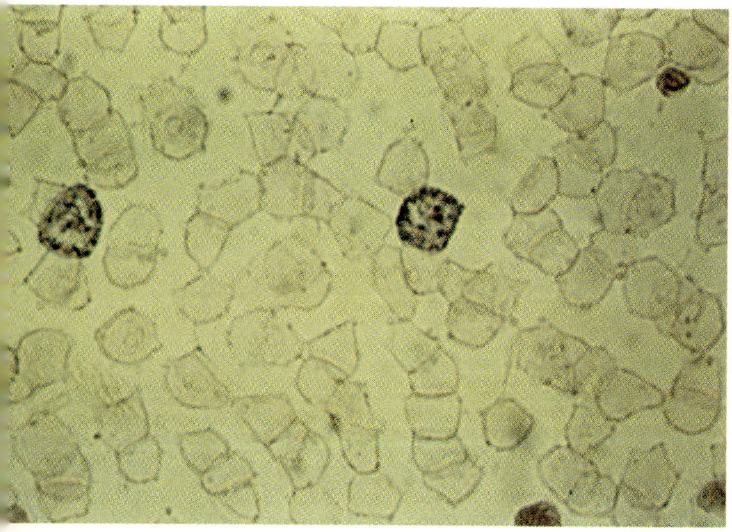

Figure 6—Feline erythrocytes with two reticulocytes (new methylene blue stain).

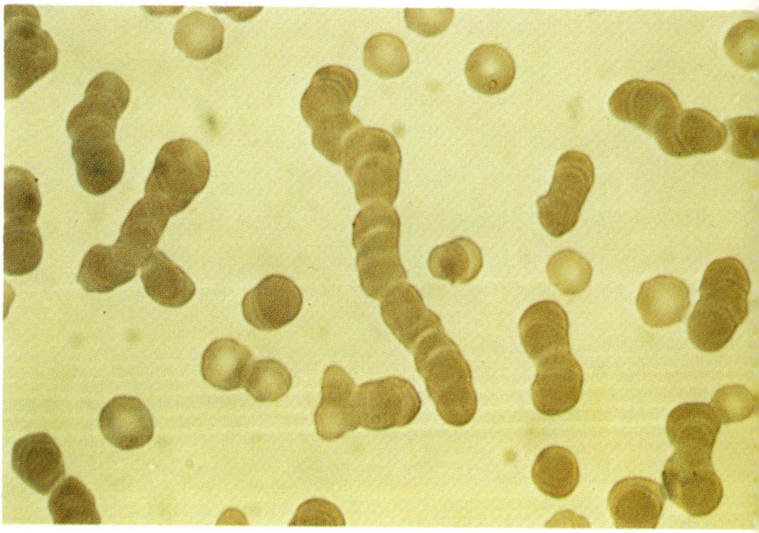

Figure 7—Equine erythrocytes with rouleau formation.

stain is allowed to age, the better the results.

Staining the blood smear

The slide is placed on a stain rack with the air-dried blood smear facing upward. If a glass cover-slip has been used for the blood smear, it can be placed on a rubber stopper or cork attached to a slide resting on the stain rack.

The blood smear is then liberally covered with the Wright's stain. If not enough stain is used, evaporation and subsequent precipitation will occur. After three to four minutes, an equal quantity

Figure 4—Feline erythrocytes with a Howell-Jolly body.

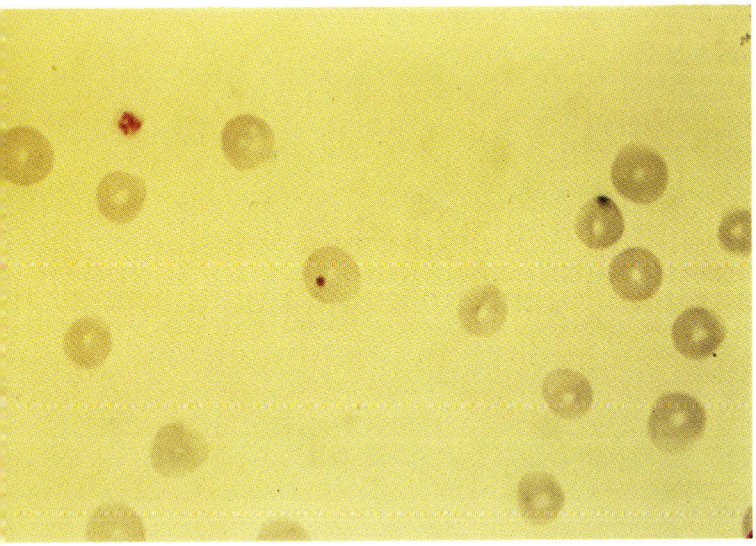

Figure 5—Feline erythrocytes with Heinz bodies (new methylene blue stain).

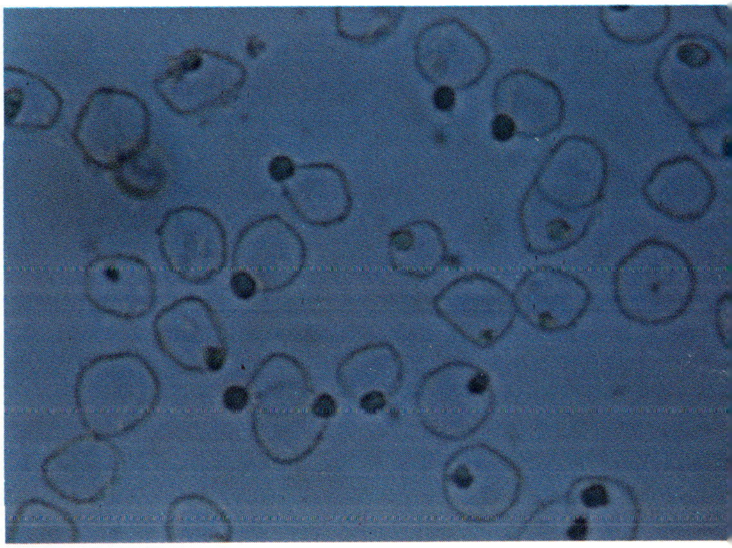

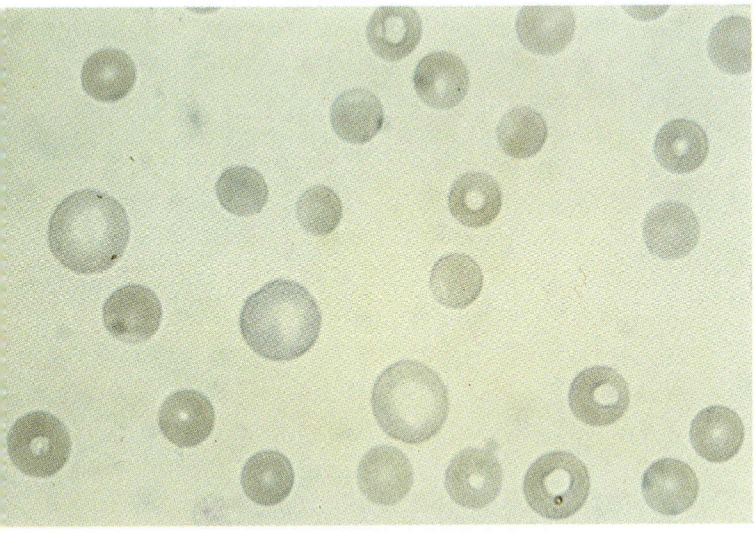

Figure 8—Canine erythrocytes with marked spherocytosis. Diagnosis: autoimmune hemolytic anemia.

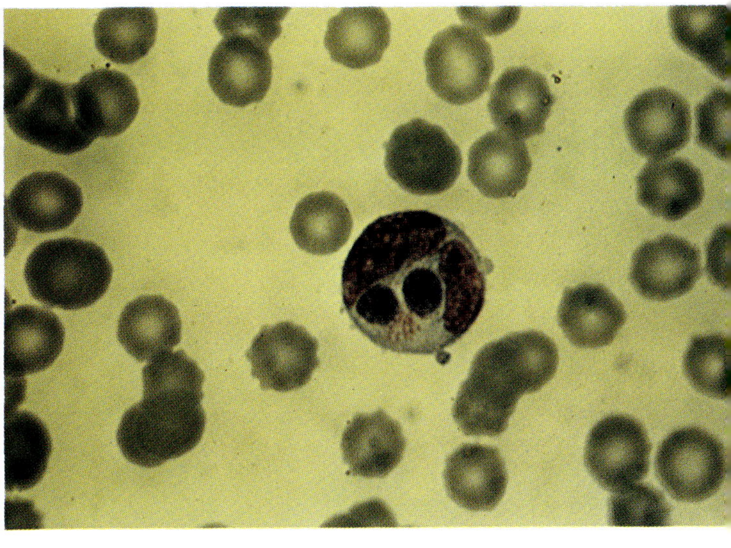

Figure 9—Canine leukocyte with *Ehrlichia canis* organism. Diagnosis: ehrlichiosis.

Figure 10—Lymphoblasts in feline peripheral blood. Diagnosis: lymphosarcoma.

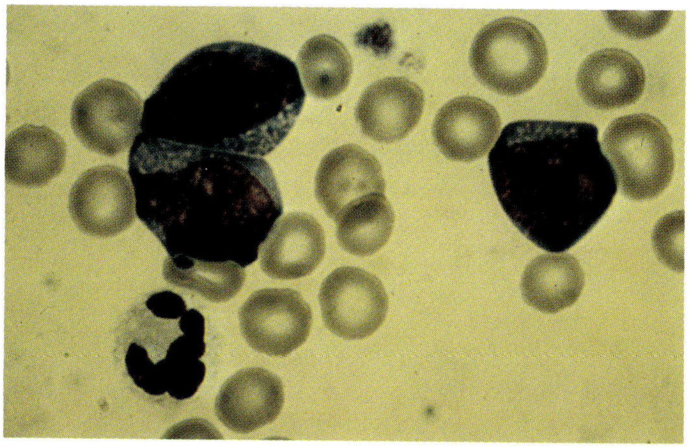

Figure 11—Monomorphic nucleated cells in feline peripheral blood. Diagnosis: myeloproliferative disease.

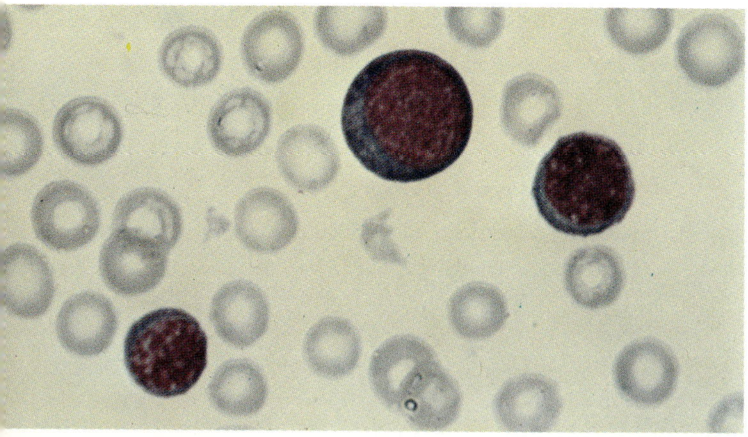

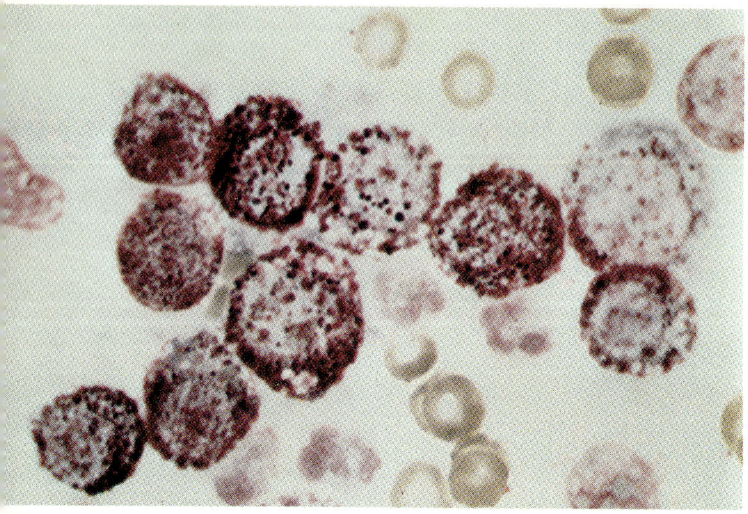

Figure 12—Feline mast cells. Diagnosis: mastosarcoma.

of buffer solution is added on top of the stain solution on the smear. A green metallic sheen should appear after the buffering solution has been added. Gentle blowing on the mixture facilitates the mixing of the buffer with the stain.

The mixture is allowed to stand for three to four minutes, then flushed off with a liberal quantity of distilled water. If the stain-buffer mixture is not liberally flushed, precipitate collects on the blood smear. The specific staining and buffering time may vary among different batches of stain.

The buffer solution used during staining is probably the most important variable in producing a well-stained blood smear. Phosphate buffers of pH 6.4 and 6.8 and plain buffered distilled water can be purchased commercially.

The specific pH of a given batch of Wright's stain usually dictates the pH of the buffer solution to be used. A couple of practice smears are made with each new batch of stain to see which buffer solution works best. If the leukocytes are understained and the erythrocytes overstained, a buffer of higher pH is needed. Conversely, if the leukocytes are overstained and the erythrocytes understained, a buffer of lower pH is needed. By trial and error with each new batch of stain, the desired staining characteristics should be achieved easily.

New methylene blue stain

New methylene blue stain is a supravital stain that stains only material containing nucleic acid; *i.e.*, leukocyte nuclei, Howell-Jolly bodies, reticulum of reticulocytes, etc. It is widely used in counting or estimating reticulocytes in anemic animals.

New methylene blue stain is available premixed or in powder form to prepare in the laboratory. The stock solution should be stored in an amber bottle, and small quantities filtered out for use. The laboratory bottle containing stain to be used should be replenished often from the stock solution, as evaporation causes loss of staining qualities.

New methylene blue stain is useful for rapidly reviewing a blood smear, as the staining procedure requires only seconds to perform. The method is simple. As soon as a drop of the stain has been applied to an unfixed, dried blood smear, the smear can be evaluated. If the smear is on a coverslip, the drop of stain is deposited on a glass slide and the coverslip smear is inverted onto the stain.

New methylene blue does not stain permanently. Therefore smears stained with new methylene blue must be studied before they dry.

Examination of the blood smear

Much valuable information can be obtained from examining a well-prepared and stained blood smear. A standard protocol should be used with every blood smear studied. This allows one to become familiar with the normals and to recognize readily the abnormals.

The first step in evaluating a blood smear should be examination under low-power magnification. With low-power magnification, the stain and the quality of the smear can be evaluated and the best areas of the smear can be identified for examination under higher magnification.

The next step is the observation of the best areas under high, dry magnification. At this magnification, the total white blood cell count (WBC) can be estimated and compared with the actual count determined by the hemocytometer or electronic cell-counter. With practice, one can become fairly adept at making gross estimates of the WBC count; this serves as a countercheck on laboratory technique. For example, if the estimated count and the determined total count differ greatly, a recheck of the total WBC count would be prudent. Generally, an average of at least three thrombocytes per high, dry field is considered adequate. Greater numbers have little significance.

With practice, one can make the differential WBC count using high, dry magnification instead of oil immersion. This significantly reduces the time required to make differential counts, because the area of vision per microscopic field is much greater.

The third step is a microscopic study of specific cell morphology under oil immersion. This step should include sequential examination of all the cellular components of the smear; *i.e.*, thrombocytes, erythrocytes, and leukocytes. Several texts on clinical hematology provide excellent photomicrographs covering specific blood cell morphology for domestic animals. *Veterinary Hematology* (Lea & Febiger) and *The Morphology of Canine and Feline Blood Cells* (Ralston Purina Co.) are notable for their reviews of blood cell morphology.

Figures 2-12 are photomicrographs illustrating some specific findings in blood smears from domestic animals.

REFERENCES

1. Davidsohn, I.; Henry, J.B.: *Clinical Diagnosis by Laboratory Methods*, 15th ed. W.B. Saunders Co., Philadelphia, Pa., 1974.
2. MacGregor, R.G.S. *et al*: The Differential Leukocyte Count. *J. Path. Bact.* *51*:337; 1940.
3. Goldston, R.T. *et al*: The Basic Clinical Pathology Laboratory—1: Selection of Equipment. *VM/SAC* *75*(1):34, 41-43; Jan. 1980.

CHAPTER 7

Anemias

ANEMIA IS A REDUCTION of the oxygen-carrying capacity of the blood that results when the hematocrit, hemoglobin, and/or total erythrocyte count fall below their normal ranges for the species. Normal ranges for the hematocrit, hemoglobin, and total erythrocyte counts for dogs and cats have been previously discussed.[1,2] Anemia, without a qualifying term (*e.g.*, iron deficiency anemia) is not a disease itself, but is a clinical sign or complication of a disease. When anemia is found, a careful evaluation of the patient's condition and a search for the underlying cause are necessary.

Anemias may be classified according to erythrocyte indices, bone-marrow responses, or pathophysiologic mechanism.[3]

Classification of anemias according to erythrocyte indices

When the erythrocyte indices are known, anemias can be classified by size (MCV), hemoglobin content (MCH), and hemoglobin concentration (MCHC) of the erythrocytes. This method of classification was originally described by Wintrobe to provide objective standards rather than subjective impressions in anemia research. The methods by which the Wintrobe erythrocyte indices are determined and the normal values for the dog and cat have been previously discussed.[2]

When this classification is used, anemias with a normal MCV are termed *normocytic*; anemias with MCV values below or above the normal ranges are termed *microcytic* or *macrocytic*, respectively, Anemias in which the MCH and MCHC are normal are termed *normochromic*; those with MCH and MCHC below normal are termed *hypochromic*. Absolute increases in hemoglobin (hyperchromasia) within erythrocytes does not occur. But increases in hemoglobin relative to the size of the erythrocyte membrane does occur, as when spherocytes are formed, as occurs with immune-mediated anemias.

The Wintrobe indices serve a useful purpose. However, as the practitioner or technician gains experience in examining properly prepared blood smears, he or she can make subjective evaluations of the erythrocytes as either microcytic or macrocytic (size), and normochromic, hypochromic, or polychromic (color). Thus, as confidence grows in making these subjective determinations, the useful-

TABLE 1—Regenerative Anemias

1. Hemorrhage (acute)
   a. Trauma
   b. Surgery
   c. G-I ulcers
   d. Warfarin toxicity
   e. Disseminated intravascular coagulation
   f. Hemophilia
2. Hemorrhage (chronic)
   a. Parasitism
   b. G-I ulcers
   c. Hematuria
   d. Hemophilia
   e. Thrombocytopenia
3. Accelerated erythrocyte destruction (hemolysis)
   a. Bacteria; *i.e.,* leptospira
   b. RBC parasites; *i.e., Haemobartonella, Babesia* spp
   c. Chemicals
      Methylene blue (feline)
      Acetaminophen (Tylenol®) (feline)
      Onion poisoning (canine)
      Phenazopyridine (feline)
   d. Immune-mediated
      Autoimmune hemolytic anemia
      Lupus erythematosis
      Blood transfusion reactions
   e. Intraerythrocytic hereditary defects
      Pyruvate kinase deficiency
      Porphyria
      Hereditary stomatocytosis
   f. Disseminated intravascular coagulation

ness of the Wintrobe erythrocyte indices becomes correspondingly less.

The methods of preparing and examining peripheral blood smears have been discussed.[4]

Classification of anemias according to response of the bone marrow

The classification of anemias according to bone-marrow response is either *regenerative* (responsive) anemia or *nonregenerative* (nonresponsive) anemia.

Regenerative anemia is seen when the bone marrow is responding by actively regenerating or producing erythrocytes (erythropoiesis). This indicates that the primary cause of the anemia has no pathologic effect on the bone marrow. The common types of regenerative anemias are those in which blood is lost (*hemorrhagic* anemia) and those in which blood is destroyed (*hemolytic* anemia).[5] The characteristic hematologic finding in cases of regenerative anemia is reticulocytosis and polychromasia. Examination of the bone marrow is not usually indicated in cases of regenerative anemia, but if the examination is performed, erythroid hyperplasia usually is seen.

Nonregenerative anemia is seen when the bone marrow cannot respond adequately to the anemia. This indicates that the primary cause of the anemia has a pathologic or suppressant effect on the bone marrow. The usual hematologic findings in cases of nonregenerative anemia are an absence of reticulocytes and no polychromasia. In nonregenerative anemias, the prognosis is generally poor. Bone-marrow examination (see subsequent chapter) is usually indicated.

Tables 1 and 2 include most regenerative and nonregenerative anemias that affect dogs and cats.

TABLE 2—Nonregenerative Anemias

1. Hypoproliferative bone marrow
   a. Chronic renal disease
   b. Endocrinopathies
      Hypothyroidism
      Hypoadrenocorticism
      Hypoandrogenism
      Hyperestrogenism
   c. Chronic disease processes
      Neoplasias
      Chronic infections
   d. Myelophthisis
      Myeloproliferative diseases
         Granulocytic leukemia
         Reticuloendothelosis
         Myelofibrosis
      Metastatic Neoplasias
   e. Infectious agents
      Feline leukemia virus
      Feline panleukopenia
      Ehrlichia canis
2. Hyperproliferative bone marrow
   a. Disorders of nucleic acid synthesis
      Vitamin B_{12} deficiency
      Folic acid deficiency
   b. Disorders of heme synthesis
      Iron deficiency anemia
      Pyridoxine deficiency
      Copper deficiency
      Lead poisoning
   c. Disorders of globin synthesis
      Erythemic myelosis
      Erythroleukemia

Classification of anemia according to pathophysiologic mechanisms

Classification of anemias on the basis of the pathophysiologic mechanisms that cause them is by 1) accelerated erythrocyte destruction (hemolytic anemias), 2) impaired erythrocyte production (aplastic anemias), or 3) blood loss (hemorrhagic anemias).

Rapidity of onset determines the clinical signs of anemia. When the onset is sudden, as in acute hemorrhage or hemolysis, pronounced signs include tachycardia, polypnea, pale mucous membranes, and possibly shock. Clinical signs may, however, be minimal (weakness, loss of stamina) or even absent if onset of anemia was gradual and the animal has adapted to the decreased oxygen-carrying capacity of the blood.

Laboratory confirmation of anemia is most easily and accurately achieved via the hematocrit. The values of the hematocrit should be interpreted in light of the animal's hydration status and any alteration caused by splenic contraction. Knowing the hemoglobin concentration and the erythrocyte count may help further classify the anemia, but those values are not usually needed to confirm the presence of anemia.

Separation of the anemias into either a regenerative or nonregenerative category is the most important step in classifying and evaluating anemias. This separation and distinction allows some prognostic latitude; *i.e.*, regenerative anemias are associated with a better prognosis than are nonregenerative anemias. This classification further reduces the diagnostic possibilities or the number of possible causes involved (*Tables 1 & 2*).

It is important to remember that in acute-onset anemias (blood loss), the signs of increased erythrocyte production or regeneration (reticulocytosis, polychromasia) will not become evident for two or three days and transfusion of whole blood may be required immediately.

Figures 1—6

Photomicrographs of blood smears showing some causes of anemias in dogs and cats that can be diagnosed by examination of the peripheral blood and the bone marrow.

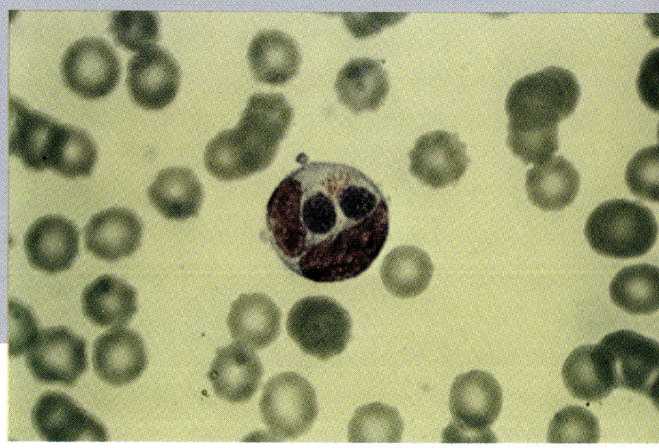

Figure 3—Canine peripheral blood (Wright stain) showing ehrlichiosis.

Regenerative anemias

Regenerative anemias suggest either a blood loss or accelerated erythrocyte destruction of sufficient magnitude and duration (two to three days) that the bone marrow responds and the peripheral blood shows reticulocytes and polychromasia.

Reticulocytosis is demonstrated by counting or estimating the number of reticulocytes in a blood smear stained with new methylene blue. The staining preparation and procedure for using new methylene blue stain have previously been discussed.[4]

The reticulocyte count is expressed as a percentage determined by differentiating 500 erythrocytes. To facilitate counting, an etched disc that divides the microscopic field into smaller squares may be inserted in one ocular (eyepiece). Examples of such discs are the Miller ocular micrometer (Bausch & Lomb for Kinsman Optical Co.) or the Net micrometer disc (American Optical, #1421A).

After the count has been completed, the percent reticulocyte count is calculated by using the formula:

$$\% \text{ reticulocyte count} = (\text{no. of reticulocytes counted} \div \text{no. of erythrocytes counted}) \times 100$$

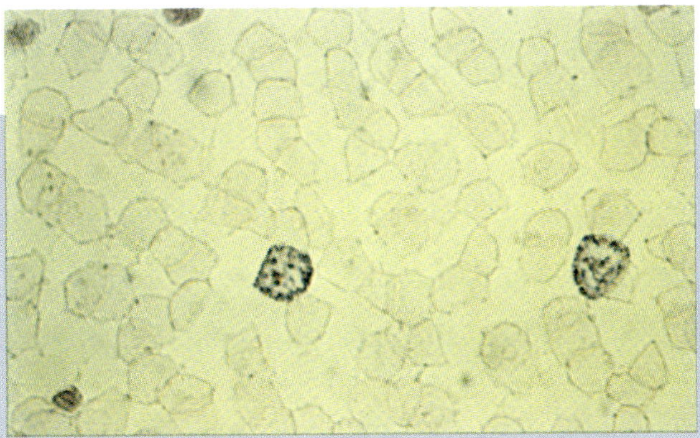

Figure 1—Feline peripheral blood (new methylene blue stain) showing reticulocytes.

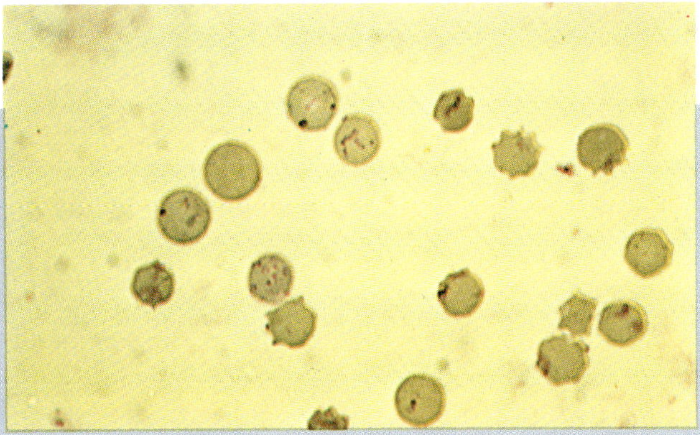

Figure 2—Feline peripheral blood (Wright stain) showing haemobartonellosis.

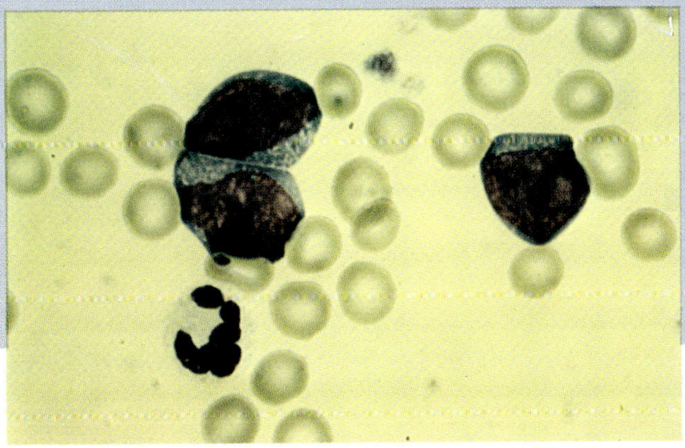

Figure 4—Feline peripheral blood (Wright stain) showing lymphosarcoma.

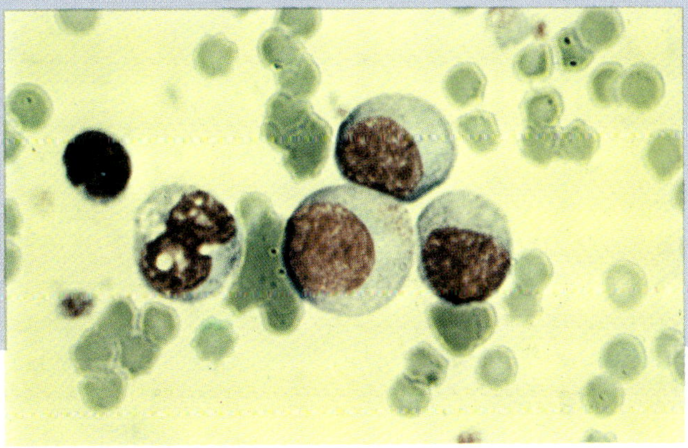

Figure 5—Feline peripheral blood (Wright stain) showing myeloproliferative disease.

With practice, the technician can subjectively estimate the number of reticulocytes by observation of a smear stained with new methylene blue.

The normal range of reticulocytes in canine blood is up to 1%. Values of 1% to 5% indicate slight regeneration, and values greater than 20% indioate marked regeneration.[6]

The amount of stained reticulum varies according to the reticulocyte's stage of maturation. Reticulocytes with heavy stippling are the *aggregate* reticulocytes; those with little stippling are the *punctate* reticulocytes. In the cat, 95% of the reticulo-

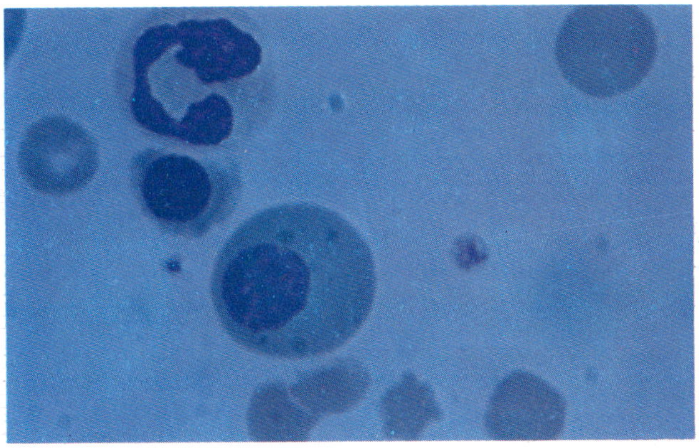

Figure 6—Feline peripheral blood (Wright stain) showing erythemic myelosis.

cytes are in the punctate form. Because of its small amount of stippling, the punctate form cannot be easily demonstrated with new methylene blue stain. For this reason, a lesser percentage of reticulocytes is seen in a cat with regenerative anemia.

The normal range of the aggregate reticulocytes in the cat is up to 0.1%. Values of 1% to 2% indicate a slight regeneration, values of 2% to 4% indicate a moderate regeneration, and values greater than 4% indicate a marked regeneration.[6]

In cases of hemorrhagic anemia, the blood loss may be external or internal, acute or chronic. With internal hemorrhage, approximately two-thirds of the erythrocytes that are lost into the body cavities are reabsorbed and returned to the circulation within three days. The other one-third of the erythrocytes are lysed or phagocytized and the iron is reused. External hemorrhage prevents reuse of the iron and plasma protein. Gastrointestinal hemorrhage is considered to be external hemorrhage.

The availability of iron determines to a great extent the magnitude of the reticulocyte response. Reticulocytosis is more pronounced in internal hemorrhage and hemolytic diseases than in external hemorrhage, due to the reuse of iron from the disrupted erythrocytes.

With chronic blood loss, the anemia develops more slowly and clinical signs are masked by the animal's adaptability to the lower oxygen-carrying capacity of the blood. A regenerative response is usual unless the iron stored in the body becomes depleted and a nonregenerative iron deficiency anemia develops. Iron deficiency anemias are characterized by serum iron levels below normal and total iron-binding capacity above normal. Normal range for serum iron levels is 75-120 μg/100 ml and normal range for iron-binding capacity is 280-340 μg/100 ml.

Iron deficiency anemia develops much more rapidly in young, fast-growing animals because they have a smaller body store of iron.

Accelerated erythrocyte destruction (hemolysis) usually has a marked regenerative response and may be accompanied by hyperbilirubinemia and icterus or hemoglobinemia.

Nonregenerative anemias

Nonregenerative anemia suggests a suppressant factor (or factors) or disease of the bone marrow that renders the marrow incapable of responding sufficiently to the anemia. Examination of the bone marrow is usually indicated in cases of nonregenerative anemia. Frequently, the examination reveals the cause of the anemia (*e.g.*, lymphosarcoma, myeloproliferative disease, etc.). The bone marrow examination also allows the anemia to be subclassified into *hypoproliferative* or *hyperproliferative* bone marrow; this division further reduces the diagnostic possibilities (*Table 2*).

A test for feline leukemia virus (FeLV) should be performed for any cat in which the cause of a nonregenerative anemia has not been diagnosed. This test is conveniently available through many commercial laboratories. A FeLV test is also marketed as an in-hospital laboratory kit (Leukassay™F—Pitman-Moore) and is relatively easy and very accurate test to determine the presence or absence of feline leukemia virus in the serum.

REFERENCES

1. Goldston, R.T. *et al*: The Basic Clinical Pathology Laboratory—3: Evaluation of the Erythrocytes: Hematocrit and Hemoglobin Determinations. *VM/SAC* 75(3):407-410; March 1980.
2. Goldston, R.T. *et al*: The Basic Clinical Pathology Laboratory—4: Evaluation of the Erythrocytes (Total Erythrocyte Count, Erythrocyte Indices, and Erythrocyte Sedimentation Rate). *VM/SAC* 75(4): 586-590; Apr. 1980.
3. Duncan, J.R.; Prasse, K.W.: *Veterinary Laboratory Medicine, Clinical Pathology*. The Iowa State University Press, Ames, Iowa, 1977.
4. Seybold, I.M. *et al*: The Basic Clinical Pathology Laboratory—5: Evaluation of the Blood Smear. *VM/SAC* 75(5):781-789; May 1980.
5. Ettinger, S.J.: *Textbook of Veterinary Internal Medicine*, Vol. 2. W.B. Saunders Co., Philadelphia, Pa., 1975.
6. Perman, V.: The Blood Smear. Notes from Central Florida Academy of Veterinary Medicine Seminar; Jan. 1980.

CHAPTER 8

Preparation of the leukocytic hemogram

CORRECT EVALUATION of leukocytes and leukocytic responses is important in clinical pathology. The leukocytic hemogram is that part of the complete blood count (CBC) dealing with the production, maturation, and possible abnormalities of leukocytes. As an integral part of the initial data base, the leukocytic hemogram consists of the total WBC count, differential cell count, and leukocytic morphology as observed in blood smears.

To evaluate leukocytes effectively, the practitioner needs a knowledge of the production, maturation, and morphologic characteristics of leukocytes. These aspects of the leukocytic series, together with interpretation, are presented in this and future articles. With knowledge of the leukocytic hemogram, important facts relating to infections, neoplastic disorders, and immunologic responses (allergic responses, etc.) can be gained. Methods of preparing and evaluating blood smears have previously been discussed.[1]

The leukocytic hemogram is acquired by observing, counting, and doing a differential tabulation of the white blood cells (leukocytes). The leukocytic series is composed of *granulocytes* and *agranulocytes*. Neutrophils, eosinophils, and basophils are granulocytes. Lymphocytes and monocytes are agranulocytes.

The blood smear should be scanned on low-power magnification (10x) to find an area where red blood cells do not overlap, but adjoin and are evenly distributed. Clumping of cells, monomorphism, blood parasites, and the quality of the stain can be determined under low-power magnification.

Under high dry magnification (100x), the number of white blood cells can be estimated. With practice, one can use this estimate to affirm that the manual or electronic white blood cell count is reasonably accurate. An average of 5 white blood cells per high dry field is found in most normal animals.[2] Although the inexperienced person should do the differential cell count on oil immersion, high dry magnification is preferred after experience has been acquired. This magnification reduces the time required to perform a differential count and gives a better overall view and relationship of the cells.

To perform the differential cell count, 200 leukocytes are counted and recorded on a cell tabulator. As the total white blood cell count increases, more cells must be differentiated. For example, a white blood cell count of 25,000/μl requires counting approximately 400 leukocytes when the differential is performed. In extreme leukopenia (*i.e.* white blood cell counts of less than 3000/μl) fewer than 200 leukocytes are adequate due to a reduced number of leukocytes on a blood smear. The differential count is best performed in a uniform, thin area of the smear. Although no specific method of counting is required for blood smears with which glass coverslips are used, a technique such as the battlement method is suggested for blood smears prepared with glass slides.[1]

The number of each type of leukocyte counted is expressed as a percentage. This percentage, multiplied by the total white blood cell count, gives the *absolute* differential cell count. The *relative* count (percentage) of any leukocyte can be elevated or depressed by a numerical change in other leukocytes. Thus, absolute values should be obtained.

If the blood smear contains nucleated red blood cells (nRBC), the total leukocyte count will be erroneously elevated since all nucleated cells are included in the total white blood cell count. When nucleated red blood cells are present in significant numbers, the number of nRBC/100 WBC should be determined when the differential cell count is performed. The total white blood cell count can be mathematically corrected by the formula:

$$\text{Corrected WBC count} = \frac{\text{Total WBC count X 100}}{100 + \text{nRBC}/100\ \text{WBC}}$$

On oil immersion, platelet adequacy can be estimated and the morphology of the erythrocytes and leukocytes can then be noted. The leukocytes should be examined for size, quantity and color of cytoplasm, granules, shape and chromatin structure of nuclei, and presence or absence of nucleoli.

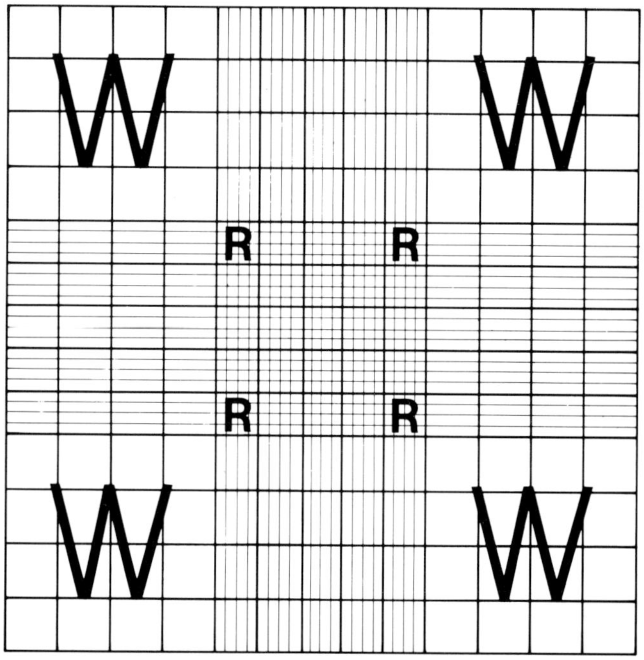

Figure 1—Erythrocyte and leukocyte counting.[3] R = zones to be counted under high-power magnification for total RBC counts. W = zones to be counted under low-power magnification for total WBC counts.

White blood cell counting

There are two basic methods of counting leukocytes in the laboratory: the hemocytometer and electronic cell counters.

The hemocytometer is the most common instrument used to derive the total white blood cell count. The hemocytometer has two ruled areas consisting of a grid of nine primary squares, each being 1 mm^2 (*Figure 1*). The four squares in the corners are subdivided into 16 squares to aid in counting white blood cells. The central square is divided into 25 squares, each of which is subdivided into 16 squares for counting red blood cells.

A regular hemocytometer leukocyte-diluting pipette or the disposable Unopette® (Becton-Dickinson) is used for measuring and diluting the cells. The Unopette system simplifies and standardizes the procedure, reducing the error of dilution for the person who uses the hemocytometer only occasionally. With this system, a capillary pipette is used to draw up a precalibrated amount of blood by capillary action. The pipetted sample is discharged into the Unopette reservoir, which contains a premeasured amount of fluid that dilutes white blood cells and lyses the erythrocytes.

When either the Unopette or the leukocyte-diluting pipette is used, the dilution factor is 1:100 and the total white blood cell count is determined by counting all the cells in the entire ruled area of the hemocytometer. The following formula is used to calculate the total white blood cell count:

Total cells in 9 squares + 10% of the total cells X 100 = WBC/μl.

Different types of Unopette reservoirs are available: sizes such as those calibrated for a 1:20 dilution and varieties such as thrombocyte-leukocyte Unopettes can be used for added convenience. Smaller diluting pipettes are also available for use with extremely high white blood cell counts; the

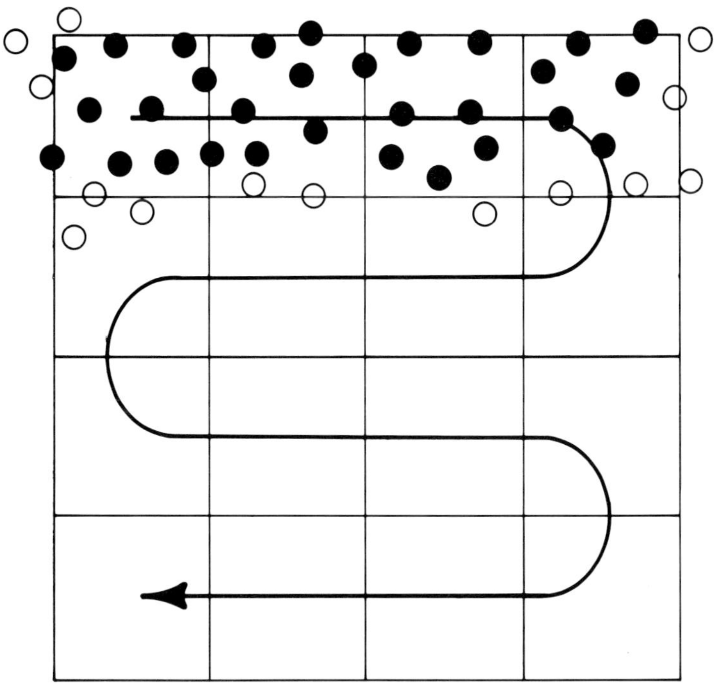

Figure 2—Leukocyte counting.[3] White blood cells touching top and left boundary lines and those within the squares are counted, alternating from left to right and right to left with succeeding horizontal rows of squares.

value obtained using these pipettes then can be multiplied by the appropriate dilution factor.

Before the hemocytometer is charged, the solution should be mixed for two minutes. The solution is then pipetted onto the edge of the platform and allowed to flow by capillary action between the chamber and coverslip. If spillage occurs, the chamber should be rinsed and the charging repeated. After the chamber is filled, the solution is placed aside for a few minutes to allow the cells to settle into a common plane.

Under low-power magnification (10x) and low illumination, the cells are counted. The procedure is to start in the upper left square and count all cells within the squares, including those cells touching the upper and left borders. A similar counting procedure is followed for each corner square. How-

Protocol for the Complete Blood Cell (CBC) Count

1. Obtain blood from animal and, if possible, make blood smears immediately. If an anticoagulant must be used, ethylene diamino tetraacetate (EDTA) is the anticoagulant of choice.
2. Fill a microhematocrit tube and centrifuge the tube to obtain packed cell volume (PCV). For dogs, check the junction of the plasma and buffy coat for microfilariae.
3. Make dilutions for a total white blood cell (WBC) count. A hemocytometer or electronic cell counter can be used to perform the total WBC count.
4. Run a red blood cell (RBC) count. An electronic cell counter is the only method recommended for this procedure due to the tremendous number of cells being counted.
5. Perform a hemoglobin determination, preferably by a photometric method; however, a color-comparison meter may be used.
6. Prepare a blood smear by either glass-slide or glass-coverslip method. Make an additional smear if the PCV is less than 30% in the dog and 25% in the cat. This smear is to be stained with new methylene blue and observed for reticulocytes. A reticulocyte count may be done with this smear. Stain the original smear with a Romanowsky-type stain (*i.e.* Wright stain).
7. On low-power magnification, scan the smear for any abnormalities, parasites, etc. Note the staining characteristics and find an area where the RBC are equally distributed for the differential count and blood cell studies.

   Proceed to high dry magnification. Estimate the WBC count and compare it with the count obtained with the hemocytometer or electronic counter. Perform a differential count, counting 200 cells. Note the number of nucleated RBCs seen/100 WBC and record.

   Proceed to oil-immersion magnification. A thorough examination is then made of the cellular morphology using a systematic protocol. This orderly study includes number and morphology of platelets, morphology of erythrocytes (size, shape, color, and inclusions), and morphology and inclusions of leukocytes.
8. Percentage of each type of leukocyte counted is multiplied by total WBC count (corrected) to obtain the absolute value for each cell type. If nucleated RBCs are seen, the WBC count must be corrected by using the formula:

$$\text{Corrected WBC count} = \frac{\text{Observed WBC count X 100}}{\text{100 + nRBC/100 WBC}}$$

   The absolute count for each leukocyte is obtained by the formula:

   Absolute count for each leukocyte =
   % of each type leukocyte X corrected total WBC count.

ever, the number of squares counted depends on the system being used (*e.g.*, with some Unopette dilutions all nine primary squares are counted). A zigzag pattern of counting the cells within the squares is used, moving from left to right and then right to left, etc. (*Figure 2*). If there is a variation of more than 15 cells between the four corner squares, the solution should be discarded and the hemocytometer recharged.

The total blood cell count is calculated by using the preceding formula or the formula recommended for the dilution used.

Electronic cell counters are becoming common in veterinary clinical laboratories. These instruments give rapid results with greater reproducibility. The factor for error is much less than that for the manual methods. The use and types of electronic counters have previously been discussed.[4]

Instructions are included with the instruments and many companies employ technical advisors who acquaint the veterinarian with the new equipment and give technical assistance in the laboratory.

The normal ranges for the total WBC count and WBC differential count for the dog and cat are presented in Table 1. Interpretation of variations in the leukocyte hemogram for the dog and cat will be covered in a subsequent article.

REFERENCES

1. Seybold, I.M. *et al*: The Basic Clinical Pathology Laboratory—5: Evaluation of the Blood Smear. *VM/SAC* 75(5):781-785, 788, 789; 1980.
2. Morgan, H.C.: Clinical Evaluation of the Blood Smear. In *Practitioner's Laboratory Manual.* Veterinary Medicine Publishing Co., Inc., Bonner Springs, Ks., 1971; pp 31-34.
3. Benjamin, M.M.: *Outline of Veterinary Clinical Pathology*, 3rd ed. Iowa State Press, Ames, Iowa, 1978.
4. Goldston, R.T. *et al*: The Basic Clinical Pathology Laboratory—4: Evaluation of the Erythrocytes (Total Erythrocyte Count, Erythrocyte Indices, and Sedimentation Rate). *VM/SAC* 75(4):586, 588-590; Apr. 1980.

TABLE 1—Ranges and Means for Leukocyte Values in the Dog and Cat*

	Dog		Cat	
Total leukocyte count (per μl)	6000—17,000 (11,500)		2500—19,500 (12,500)	
	per μl	percentage	per μl	percentage
Segmented neutrophil	3000—11,500 (7000)	60—77 (70)	2500—12,500 (7500)	35—75 (59)
Band neutrophil	0—300 (70)	0—3 (0.8)	0—300 (100)	0—3 (0.5)
Lymphocyte	1000—4800 (2800)	12—30 (20)	1500—7000 (4000)	20—55 (32)
Eosinophil	100—1250 (550)	2—10 (4)	0—1500 (650)	2—12 (5)
Basophil	Rare	Rare	Rare	Rare
Monocyte	150—1350 (750)	3—10 (5)	0—850 (350)	1—4 (3)

*Reprinted in part from Ettinger, S.J.: *Textbook of Veterinary Internal Medicine,* Vol. 2. W.B. Saunders Co., Philadelphia, Pa., 1975.

CHAPTER 9

Evaluation of the leukocytes:

morphology, production, maturation, and function

CLINICAL evaluation of abnormalities and diseases relating to leukocytes is routine to most in-hospital laboratories. This evaluation should include both quantitative and qualitative measurements (differential and total WBC counts and morphology). A change from the expected norms in either the number or morphology of leukocytes will either give a diagnosis or direct the practitioner to other diagnostic aids. Accurate interpretation of leukocyte response requires knowledge of the function, production, distribution, and fate of leukocytes. These aspects of normal leukocytes will be discussed in this series on the leukocytic hemogram.

Production and maturation of leukocytes occurs in an orderly manner. The process of granulopoiesis begins when a pluripotential stem cell gives rise to the unipotential myeloblast. The unipotential myeloblasts develop progressively into progranulocytes, myelocytes, metamyelocytes (juveniles), band cells, and segmented cells (*Figures 1-5*). Progranulocytes give rise to neutrophilic, eosinophilic, or basocytophilic myelocytes. This is known as the Schilling maturation process (*Figure 6*).[1]

Agranulocytes, which include lymphocytes and monocytes, are not produced in the same manner as cells of the granulocytic series. The lymphocyte is produced from embryonic stem cells that seed the thymus and bursa-equivalent lymphoid tissue (gut-associated lymphoid tissue or bone marrow) in the embryo. Monocytes probably originate from stem cells in the bone marrow and begin migrating, via the bloodstream, into the tissues where they are known as *tissue macrophages*.

Morphology

The leukocytes comprising the granulocytic series originate from the unipotential cell, the myeloblast. The myeloblast is a round cell, 15 μ to 20 μ in diameter. The nucleus is round-to-oval with purple, evenly dispersed chromatin and one or two prominent nucleoli.

Progranulocytes develop from the myeloblast and are slightly larger than the myeloblast. The eccentrically situated nucleus of the progranulocyte begins to clump and the nucleolus becomes less obvious as the maturation process continues. The cytoplasm is abundant and contains nonspecific azurophilic granules. Progranulocytes rarely appear in the peripheral blood. Normally, the bone marrow contains few myeloblasts or progranulocytes.

The next cell, the myelocyte, can be differentiated on the basis of its specific granules into a neutrophilic, eosinophilic, and basocytophilic cell. The myelocyte is slightly smaller in diameter than the myeloblast and progranulocyte. The cytoplasm of the myelocyte is pale blue and contains specific granules. The nucleus is oval, eccentric, and has no nucleoli. Significant numbers of neutrophilic myelocytes are in the bone marrow but rarely are found in peripheral blood. The myelocytic stage is the last stage in which cell division occurs.

The three different types of myelocytes then develop into metamyelocytes. Moderate numbers of neutrophilic metamyelocytes are in the bone marrow. In severe left-shift neutrophilias, large numbers of metamyelocytes appear in the peripheral blood. As maturation progresses, metamyelocytes become smaller but do not divide. The nucleus is bean-shaped and the cytoplasm is pale gray. The cytoplasmic granules of the neutrophilic metamyelocyte still are difficult to see.

The bone marrow contains many band neutrophils and a few are found in the peripheral blood of healthy dogs and cats. The nucleus is smooth and usually appears as a U- or an S-shaped curve. Stained with Wright stain, the cytoplasm is pale gray with pale-colored granules. When stained with new methylene blue, the cytoplasmic granules are not clearly seen. Differentiation of cells on the basis of nuclear morphology is of value when water-soluble stains such as new methylene blue are used.

Many segmented neutrophils are found in the bone marrow; they are the most numerous leukocyte in the dog and cat.[2] They are slightly larger in diameter than the erythrocyte. Their nucleus usually has two lobes. Those with more than four lobes are considered abnormal. These abnormal neutrophils, labeled *hypersegmented*, indicate a right shift. Chromatin clumps and irregular nuclear membranes are considered normal. A small appendage, the Barr body, may be found attached to the nucleus (*Figure 5*). This body is the sex chromatin in female dogs and cats.

The two other granulocytes, eosinophils and basophils, go through a maturation series similar to that of the neutrophil.

The eosinophilic and basocytophilic series are easy to identify by their specific granules. Eosinophilic granules stained with Romanovsky stains are pale orange to bright red. In dogs, the granules are round, vary in size, and do not fill the cytoplasm (*Figure 7*). In cats, the granules are rod-shaped, pale red, and of uniform size (*Figure 8*).

Canine basophils are large cells that have dark basophilic cytoplasmic granules outlined by a gray cytoplasm (*Figure 9*). These granules are water-soluble and may not be visible under staining with new methylene blue. Feline basophils contain round, lavender granules (*Figure 10*).

Figure 1—Progranulocyte (dog).

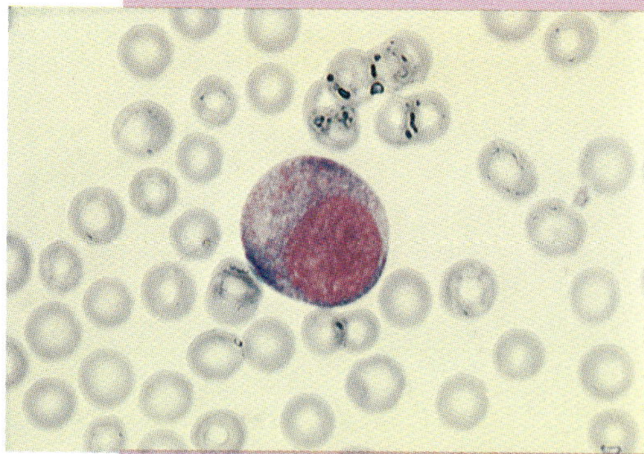

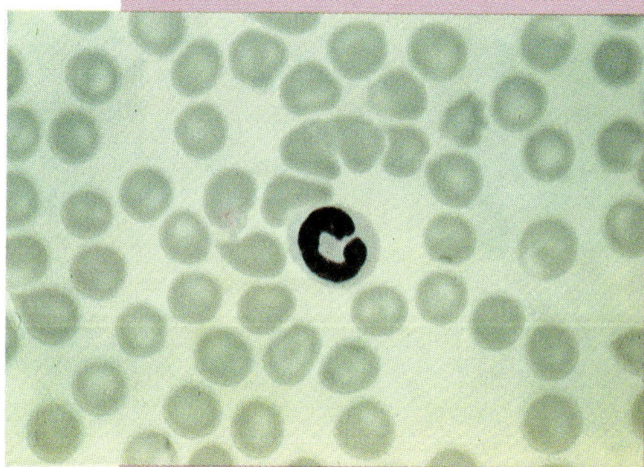

Figure 4—Band neutrophil (dog).

Lymphocytes are round, with a nucleus that almost fills the interior of the cell. Populations of large and small lymphocytes, in which small lymphocytes predominate, are found in dogs and cats. The nucleus of small lymphocytes is deep blue-black with a narrow rim of cytoplasm (*Figure 11*). Large lymphocytes are smooth with coarsely arranged, purple nuclear chromatin (*Figure 12*). Small lymphocytes require differentiation from metarubricytes in cases of regenerative anemia.

Figure 2—Myelocyte (dog).

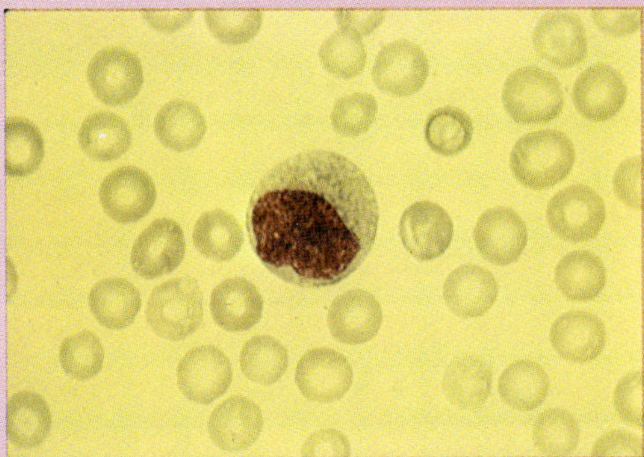

Figure 3—Metamyelocyte (dog).

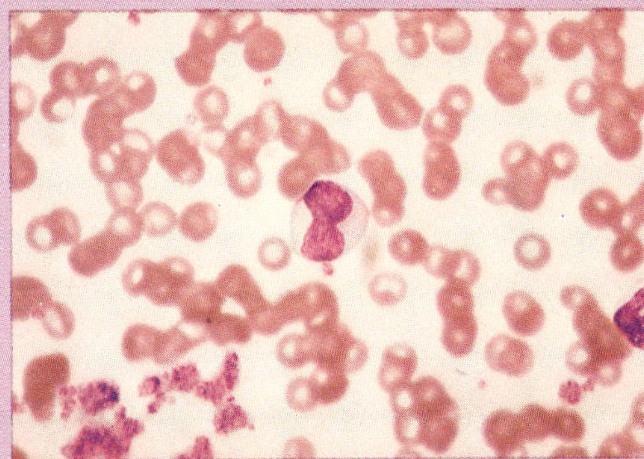

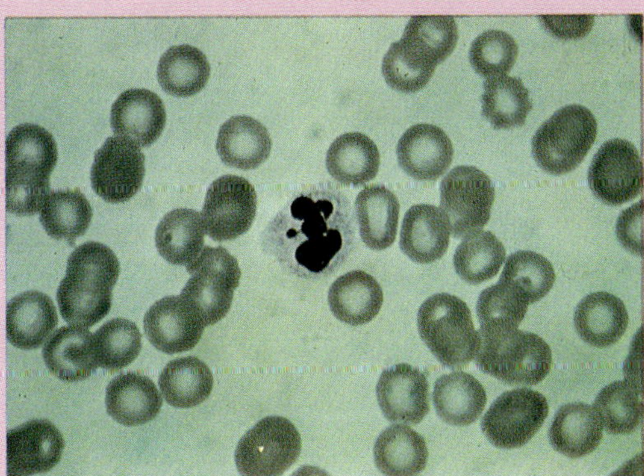

Figure 5—Segmented neutrophil with Barr body (dog).

Compared to small lymphocytes, metarubricytes have densely aggregated chromatin within a round, darker-staining nucleus. The nuclear:cytoplasmic ratio is less in the metarubricyte and the cytoplasm is slightly orange.

Monocytes, the largest blood leukocytes, have a blue-gray cytoplasm that is frequently vacuolated. Their nuclei vary in size and shape (*Figure 13*). The nucleus can be oval, bean-shaped, trilobular, or slightly elongated, and has chromatin arranged in strands or lace-like patterns. These features can

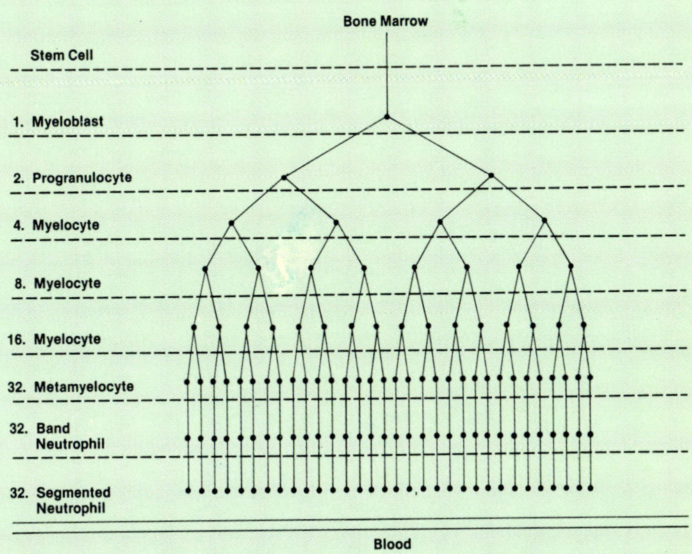

Figure 6 The Schilling maturation process of leukocytes.

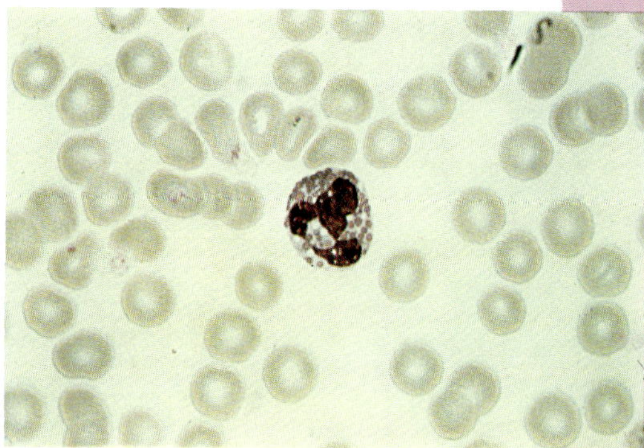

Figure 7—Canine eosinophil.

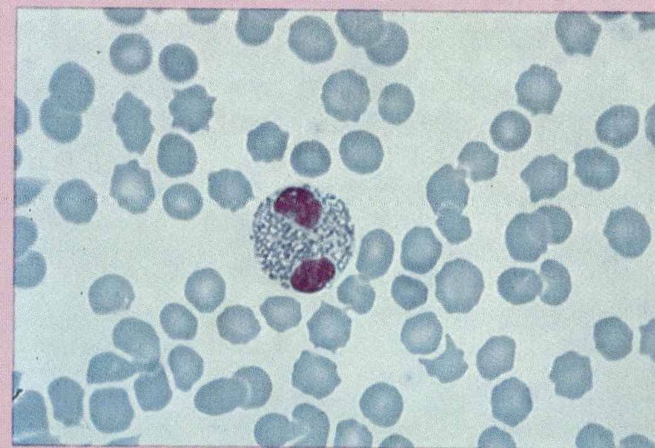

Figure 8—Feline eosinophil.

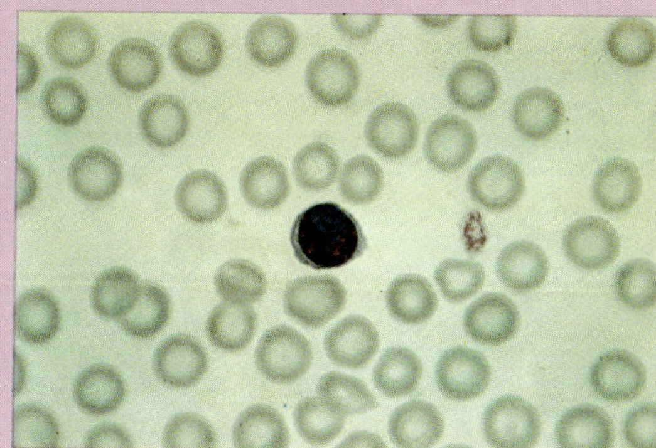

Figure 11—Small lymphocyte (dog).

be used to differentiate monocytes from large lymphocytes which have smooth nuclear chromatin, and from neutrophilic metamyelocytes which have evenly dispersed nuclear clumps. In aged blood, monocytes may become more vacuolated.

Production and maturation

Neutrophils are considered to have four pools containing cells of different ages: 1) the proliferating pool, 2) the maturation pool, 3) the marginal pool, and 4) the circulating pool (*Figure 14*).

The proliferating pool, centered in the bone marrow, contains myeloblasts, progranulocytes, and myelocytes. Myeloblasts divide once, progranulocytes twice, and myelocytes four or more times.[1]

The maturation pool, also found in the bone marrow, contains cells that do not divide but mature from metamyelocytes to band and segmented neutrophils. Neutrophils comprise 60% to 77% of all circulating blood leukocytes in the dog and 35% to 75% in the cat. Normal values for the dog and cat have been listed elsewhere.[3]

The marginal neutrophilic pool is found along the walls of capillaries and postcapillary venules. These cells move more slowly than the neutrophils in the circulating pool. In the cat the marginal pool is 70% larger than the circulating pool.[1,4] Excitation of the animal can cause mobilization of a tremendous number of cells from the marginal pool into the circulating pool.

Neutrophils in the circulating pool are those normally found in total and differential cell counts. They have a half life of 6 to 7 hours. The entire population is replaced every 60 hours. These cells

Figure 9—Canine basophil *(right)* and segmented neutrophil *(left)*.

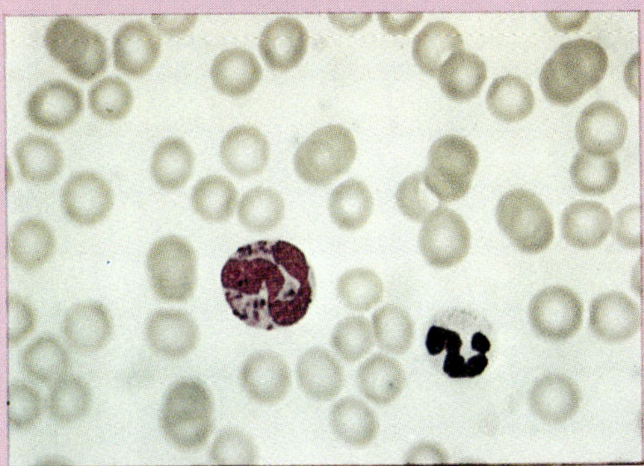

Figure 10—Feline basophil *(left)* and segmented neutrophil *(right)*.

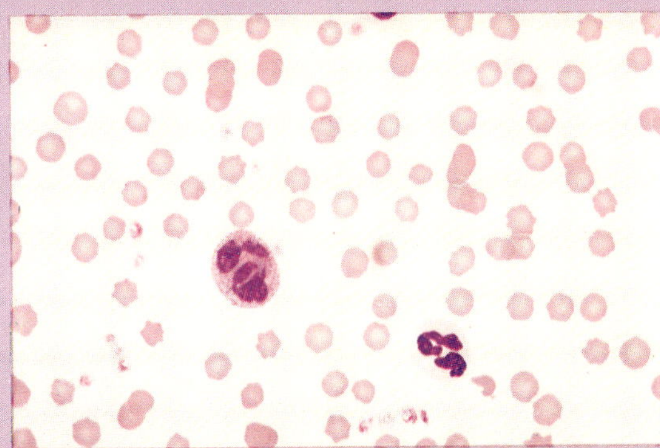

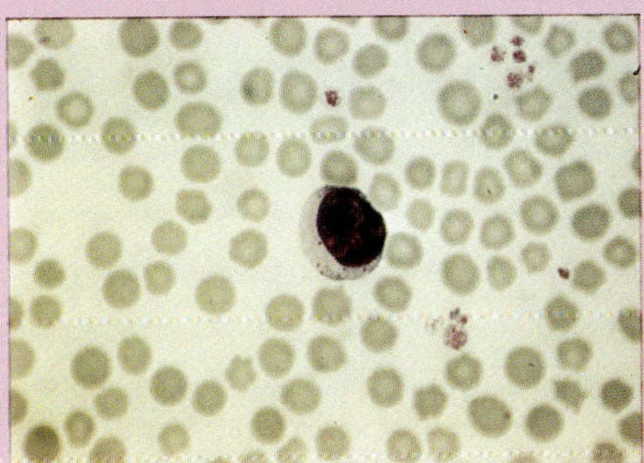

Figure 12—Large lymphocyte (cat).

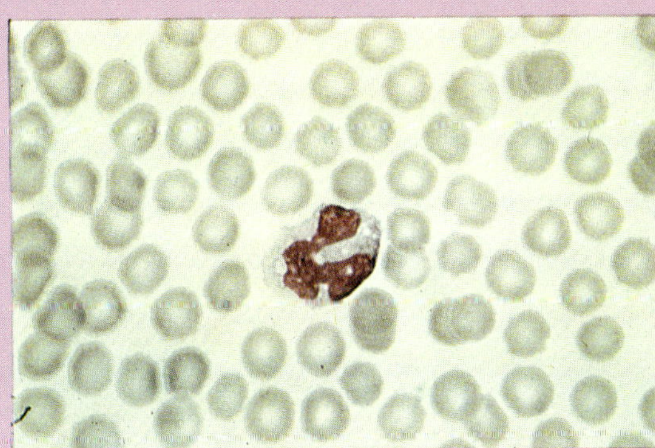

Figure 13—Monocyte (dog).

are normally lost into tissues and are found in many body secretions.

In response to inflammation, neutrophils are released from the storage or marginal pool within a few hours after the inciting cause. Reduced attrition and accelerated production of cells occurs in 3 to 4 days and an increase in stem-cell production occurs in five days. All of these events have an effect on the number of neutrophils in the blood.

A left shift results when immature neutrophils are found in the peripheral blood. Frequently, in the dog, left shifts are found with many bands and metamyelocytes, whereas in the cat a left shift seldom contains any cells less mature than bands.

Left-shift neutrophilias fall into *regenerative* and *degenerative* categories. With a regenerative left shift there is a slight-to-moderate increase in immature neutrophils in the peripheral blood, together with an elevated WBC count. With a degenerative left shift, the WBC count is normal or less than normal.

In a right-shift neutrophilia, the nuclei of the neutrophils become hypersegmented (more than four segments) due to aging. Excessive contact time with anticoagulants causes neutrophils to become hypersegmented. Corticosteroids, which inhibit diapedesis, also cause increased aging and hypersegmentation of these cells.

Eosinophils and basophils originate in the bone marrow and follow a maturation process similar to that of neutrophils. Usually the bone marrow contains 300 to 400 eosinophils for each one in circulation. Eosinophils are sequentially released from the bone marrow, circulate for a certain length of time, and migrate into the tissues of the body. These cells, like neutrophils and basophils, do not return to the circulation. The number of basophils appears to be inversely related to the number of mast cells in connective tissue. Cats have few basophils but many mast cells, whereas rabbits have many basophils and few mast cells.[1]

Lymphocytes arise from the thymus or bursa-equivalent lymphoid tissue (gut-associated lymphoid tissue or bone marrow). In the embryo, stem

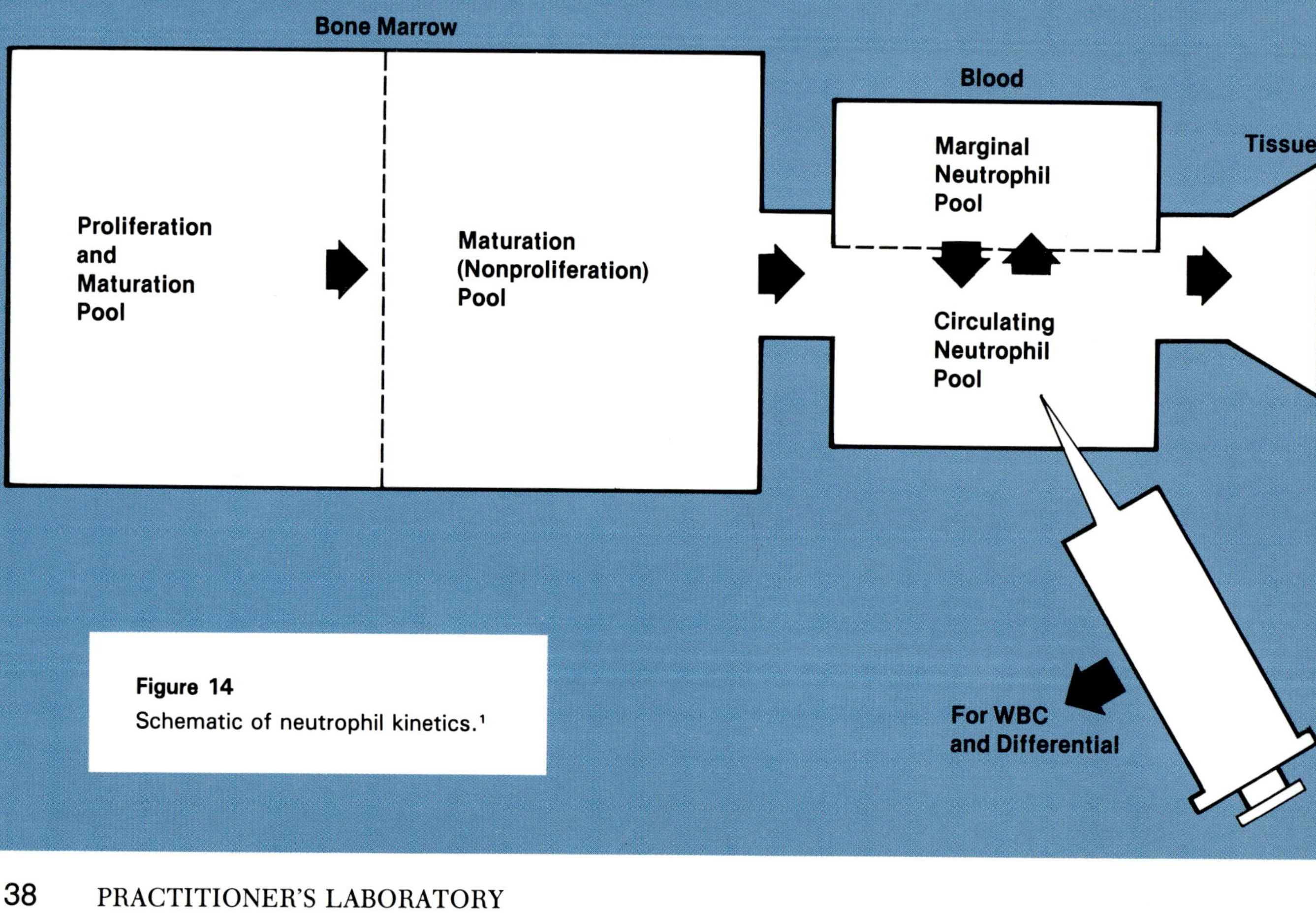

Figure 14
Schematic of neutrophil kinetics.[1]

cells seed these areas. Two fundamentally different populations of lymphocytes arise: T-lymphocytes from the thymus lymphoid tissue and B-lymphocytes from the bursa-equivalent lymphoid tissue. These cells are conditioned for certain responses that relate to humoral and cell-mediated immunity.

Lymphocytes can be classified into long- or short-lived cells. The long-lived lymphocytes live for months to years and retain the ability to divide. These constitute the bulk of cells in the blood, lymph-node cortex, and the white pulp of the spleen. They are responsive to antigenic stimulation. The short-lived lymphocytes live for 1 to 3 days and are found mainly in the thymus and bone marrow. One important difference of lymphocytes from other leukocytes is their ability to recirculate.

The exact origin of monocytes is not certain, but most authorities agree that they probably are produced in the bone marrow.[5] In man, the distribution of monocytes parallels that of neutrophils, with the marginal pool being five times larger than the circulating pool.[1] Monocytes migrate through the bloodstream into body tissues, where they become macrophages and phagocytize dead or damaged cells.

Function

Neutrophils function in inflammatory and phagocytic conditions. The products of bacterial and tissue breakdown are the major chemotactic agents that cause neutrophils to marginate and migrate through endothelial openings in blood vessels and aggregate near an agent.[6] Phagocytosis occurs at this time. Bacteria or other tissues are ingested and broken down by digestive enzymes contained in lysosomes of the neutrophil. Cells less mature than metamyelocytes cannot phagocytize.

Eosinophils are attracted to areas of the body by release of histamine. Histamine release occurs after tissue is disrupted. Mast cells and basophils, which contain histamine, degranulate when they are subjected to injury or lymphokine (antigen-antibody) reactions. Eosinophils phagocytize and detoxify foreign substances and decomposed body protein. The role of eosinophils in antigen-antibody reactions is not fully known, but when histamine is released in conjunction with most antigen-antibody reactions, eosinophils are almost always present.

Basophils are produced in the bone marrow and have a life expectancy of 10 to 12 days. Mast cells are the connective-tissue counterpart of basophils which are located in peripheral blood. Mast cells differ in having a round nucleus and stellate-to-round granules. The granules are delicate and usually more numerous.

The lysosomes of the basophil contain heparin, histamine, serotonin, and hyaluronic acid which can be easily released. Injury to tissue can cause the release of histamine and serotonin, inciting an inflammatory response. This inflammatory response increases capillary permeability and the attraction of eosinophils. Heparin, a potent anticoagulant, probably prevents blood and lymph from coagulating around the exudates.

Basophils are involved in cellular immunity, with antigenic stimulation initiating their increased production. Basophils have been implicated in both immediate and delayed hypersensitivities. Antibodies bound to the cellular membrane of the basophil can cause lysis if they combine with an antigen.

The bone marrow provides stem cells that seed the thymus and bursa-equivalent lymphoid tissue in the embryo. These cells give rise to the two fundamental types of lymphocytes:[6] 1) T or thymic-dependent lymphocytes which initiate cell-mediated immunity and 2) B or bursa-equivalent lymphocytes which produce antibodies and are the precursors of plasma cells. Plasma cells are the main cellular source of antibodies (immunoglobins). Thymic-dependent lymphocytes are located in the deep cortex of lymph nodes, spleen, thoracic duct, and thymus. B-cells are found as precursors in the bone marrow and germinal center of lymphocytes. Most circulating lymphocytes are T-lymphocytes.

The majority of lymphocytes live for years. These cells circulate for about two hours before returning through the postcapillary venules. Usually, there is a constant number of lymphocytes that gradually decreases as the animal ages. T and B cells cannot be distinguished from one another under the microscope. Microscopically, lymphocytes can be classified only as small or large cells.

Cell-mediated immunity (T-lymphocytes) is involved in delayed hypersensitivities, tuberculin-type reactions, contact dermatitis, and autoimmune reactions. Humoral immunity (B-lymphocytes) is involved with anaphylactic reactions, allergies, virus and toxin neutralizations, and immune-complex diseases.

Monocytes originating in the bone marrow transform into tissue macrophages, constituting the reticuloendothelial system. Macrophages live for about 100 days. They function late in the course of inflammatory lesions, phagocytizing foreign material and dead cells. Monocytes appear in the recovery stages of chronic pyogenic bacterial infections and are involved in processing antigenic information. Although the reticuloendothelial system is involved with body defenses, it is not as responsive as neutrophils to blood-borne pyogenic infections.

REFERENCES

1. Prasse, K.W.: Disorders of the Leukocytes. In *Textbook of Internal Medicine*, Vol. II. W.B. Saunders, Philadelphia, Pa., 1975; pp 1627-1660.
2. Schalm, O.W. *et al*: *Veterinary Hematology*, 3rd ed. Lea & Febiger, Philadelphia, Pa., 1975.
3. Wilkes, R.D. *et al*: The Clinical Pathology Laboratory—7: Preparation of the Leukocytic Hemogram. *VM/SAC* 75(7):1101-1107; 1980.
4. Raab, S.O. *et al*: Granulokinetics in Normal Dogs. *Am. J. Physiol.* *206*:83; 1964.
5. Schmalzl, F. *et al*: On the Origin of Monocytes. *Acta Haematol.* (Basal) 39:117; 1968.
6. Benjamin, M.M.: *Outline of Veterinary Clinical Pathology*, 3rd ed. Iowa State Univ. Press, Ames, Iowa, 1979; p 81.

CHAPTER 10

Interpretation of the leukocytic hemogram

THE EVALUATION OF LEUKOCYTES should include quantitative total and differential white blood cell (WBC) counts, and subjective observations of morphology. The interpretation of these changes seldom provides a diagnosis, but it becomes important when combined with history and clinical signs. The elevation or depression of leukocytes is referred to as leukocytosis and leukopenia, respectively.

Neutrophilia

Neutrophilia can result from either physiologic or pathologic changes. It is the usual cause of leukocytosis. The degree of neutrophilia depends on the cause and severity of the disease, resistance of the animal, whether the infection is localized or generalized, therapy, and the animal species involved. A neutrophil count greater than 11,500/μl in the dog and 12,500/μl in the cat is a neutrophilia.[1]

Noninflammatory

With physiologic neutrophilia, total WBC counts are greater than normal without the presence of disease. This condition occurs with increased exercise or the release of epinephrine caused by fear or excitement. Release of endogenous epinephrine mobilizes all leukocytes, especially neutrophils, from the marginal pool into the circulating pool. During physiologic neutrophilia there is usually no increased movement of leukocytes from the bone marrow to the circulation or from the circulation to the body tissues. A very slight left shift may occur. Physiologic neutrophilia occurs frequently in healthy cats and WBC counts can reach 20,000 to 30,000/μl. A WBC count of this magnitude, accompanied by a possible lymphocytosis and a slight, if any, left shift, is a good indication of a physiologic leukocytosis. Dogs can have a mild physiologic neutrophilia postprandially and during pregnancy.

Frequently, noninflammatory neutrophilia results from trauma, intoxication, convulsions, neoplasia, certain metabolic and endocrine disorders, surgical manipulations, or anesthesia. These are all sources of systemic stress. Stress initiates the release of endogenous corticosteroids which mobilize marginal-pool neutrophils, increase release of neutrophils from the bone marrow, and increase the half-life of the neutrophil by prolonging the neutrophil's period of circulation. These changes cause the number of blood neutrophils to increase one to five times, with a slight left shift. The use of corticosteroids and adrenocorticotropic hormone (ACTH) can cause a similar neutrophilia.

If exogenous glucocorticoids are given or stress occurs, the neutrophilic response occurs within a few hours and returns to normal within 24 hours. The duration of the response to exogenous glucocorticoids is dose-dependent. A small number of neutrophils will become hypersegmented because of the prolonged circulation time. Repeating the leukogram helps confirm this type of neutrophilia.

Lymphopenia and eosinopenia have been used to differentiate stress-induced neutrophilias from inflammatory disorders. However, stress can occur in both inflammatory and noninflammatory disorders. Monocytosis occurs with stress in dogs and cats. Basopenia occurs with stress in dogs only.[2] Toxic neutrophils would rule out a diagnosis of noninflammatory neutrophilia.

A hemolytic crisis can produce a greater neutrophilic leukocytosis and a significant left shift.

Inflammatory

Inflammation is the cellular or humeral response to tissue injury. It is one of the more important reasons for evaluating leukocytes. The clinical course of an inflammatory disease can be followed by repeated examination of the leukocytes.

Inflammatory neutrophilias result from bacteria, viruses, fungi, and other infectious agents. Noninfectious agents, such as chemicals or heat, may also cause an inflammatory neutrophilia. Local inflammatory conditions and pyogenic organisms produce higher neutrophil levels than do generalized or nonpyogenic infections.

As demand by the tissues for neutrophils increases, some unknown stimulus acts on the bone marrow to increase granulopoiesis. A chemical similar to erythropoietin (stimulus for production of red blood cells) is believed to exist for the production of WBCs. This chemical or compound is known as granulopoietin. The number of neutrophils found on a cell count depends on the balance between the demand for neutrophils by the tissues and the production of neutrophils in bone marrow.

In cases of acute inflammation, neutrophils in the marginal pool enter the circulating pool which, in turn, stimulates the bone marrow. If the production and release of neutrophils by the bone marrow exceeds the demand of tissues for neutrophils, a neutrophilic leukocytosis occurs with a regenerative left shift. A degenerative left shift occurs when production or release cannot satisfy tissue demand. This excessive demand or failure of production can lead to a neutropenia and a grave prognosis. Chronic inflammation or localized suppuration can produce marked left shifts represented by numerous band and metamyelocytic neutrophils. When repeated WBC counts indicate similar blood values, the peak of inflammation has occurred,

The magnitude of neutrophilic leukocytosis roughly parallels the magnitude of inflammation. In dogs and cats, the majority of neutrophilic leukocytoses falls within a range of 20,000 to 30,000 WBC/μl.[3] Pyelonephritis, neoplasia, distemper, or secondary bacterial infection frequently produce these values in dogs. Common causes in cases of severe infection (30,000 to 50,000 WBC/μl) are pyometra, pyogenic abscesses, pleuritis, pneumonia, endocarditis, and leptospirosis.[1] Intense suppuration is suspected when the number of immature neutrophils equals or exceeds that of segmented neutrophils. Excessive release of corticosteroid or exhaustion of granulopoiesis may result in a degenerative left shift. A declining or minimal left shift in the presence of clinical illness is basis for an unfavorable prognosis. Such chronic problems as severe pyoderma, bacterial endocarditis, and pyometra are examples of this situation.

Neutropenia

Neutropenia, a deficiency of neutrophils in the peripheral blood, is always associated with leukopenia in dogs and cats. A grave prognosis often accompanies an absolute neutropenia.

Excessive destruction or utilization of neutrophils occurs with overwhelming bacterial infections, certain viral diseases, and hypersplenism. Acute peritonitis, aspiration pneumonia, and acute suppurative metritis are examples of infections that result in excessive demand for neutrophils by tissues. This increased demand results in a shortened neutrophil half-life and a degenerative left shift. Toxic neutrophils are frequently seen during the course of severe inflammatory disease induced by systemic toxemia. The degenerative left shift may contain band, metamyelocytic, and myelocytic neutrophils. Bizarre and giant cell forms may be seen. In most neutropenias, the prognosis should be withheld until repeat examinations of leukocytes can be completed. At that time, an increasing neutrophil count, even when it still is considered a degenerative left shift, may be reason for a more favorable prognosis.

Sequestration of neutrophils can occur by margination in capillary beds, or can occur secondarily to anaphylactic or endotoxic shock. Sequestration is usually followed by a leukocytosis.

Reduced granulopoiesis commonly occurs with chronic infections, administration of certain drugs, and malignancies. These diseases are serious and their diagnosis usually requires other clinical and laboratory findings.

In gray Collies, a condition known as *cyclic neutropenia* occurs. It is manifested as a profound neutropenia followed by a cyclic resurgence of neutrophils. An increase in serum muramidase action precedes a rise in WBC count. The cycle has intervals of 8 to 12 days and is lethal in both sexes.[2]

The mechanism by which a virus induces neutropenia is not understood. The neutropenia usually is mild, transient, and followed by a neutrophilic leukocytosis. This leukocytosis probably results from secondary bacterial infection. A regenerative left shift accompanies the leukocytosis. The upper respiratory disease complex in cats does not involve a classical virus-induced neutropenia as would be expected. A low neutrophil count accompanies canine distemper and infectious canine hapatitis early in the disease; a mild neutrophilia develops later.

Feline panleukopenia extremely depresses bone marrow production, resulting in a profound neutropenia, with only lymphocytes and a few immature neutrophils in the blood. On subsequent leukograms a rising neutrophil count could indicate the recovery phase of the infection. With this disease the left shift may not be orderly, and bizarre neutrophilic forms may be present. Leukemia should not be diagnosed when erratic-appearing neutrophils are seen in the blood of a cat during the first few days of recovery from panleukopenia.[1]

Systemic toxemia, especially from exotoxin-producing bacteria, causes morphologic changes in neutrophils that can be used as a prognostic tool. Neutrophilic changes usually are severe enough to require a guarded prognosis. Morphologic changes should be recorded with the differential cell count.

The mildest toxic change is the inclusion of Dohle bodies in the cytoplasm of neutrophils. These bodies are blue, angular granules that result from minor abnormalities in the cytoplasmic maturation process. A more severe change results in large neutrophils with a faintly basophilic, foamy cytoplasm. The abnormalities used in determining the degree of toxicity are cytoplasmic foaminess, vacuolization, cell size, and degree of basophilia.

Recovery from depressed granulopoiesis and anemias caused by a deficiency of vitamin B_{12} or folic acid may give rise to neutrophils with asynchronous nuclear and cytoplasmic maturation. The result is giant cells and binucleated cells.[3] Care should be taken not to diagnose a neoplastic disorder on the basis of these changes.

Eosinophilia and eosinopenia

Eosinophilia and eosinopenia occur often among dogs and cats. Eosinophilia is associated with allergic and parasitic disorders, but the response may be inconsistent. In dogs, eosinophilia occurs when blood values exceed 1200 cells/μl. The tissue affected, the duration of exposure to tissue irritants, the magnitude of tissue injury, the nature of the irritant, and the presence or absence of antigenic stimulation will influence the degree of eosinophilia.[1] An eosinophilia often is associated with allergies, eosinophilic pneumonia, eosinophilic gastroenteritis, heartworm and other parasitic diseases, adrenocortical insufficiency, and proestrus.[2]

Any agent that incites degranulation of mast cells and release of histamine enhances eosinophilia. Mechanical agents include such biologic substances as bacterial toxins, snake venoms, and leukocyte lysosomes. Physical agents include heat, ultraviolet light, and x-rays. Antibody-antigen reactions involving mast cells can cause release of histamine. A greater eosinophilia is expected with subsequent exposure to an agent.

Eosinophilia is most often associated with skin conditions, followed in order of incidence by respiratory problems, parasites, and inflammatory conditions of the gastrointestinal tract.[1] Eosinophilic enterocolitis occurs mainly in German Shepherd dogs. In dogs, estrus can cause a transient eosinophilia. Canine dirofilariasis and certain neoplasia also can produce eosinophilia. Adrenal insufficiency is usually associated with eosinophilia.

In many diseases, the eosinophil count of cats parallels that of dogs. An eosinophilia often occurs in cases of eosinophilic granuloma, aelurostrongylosis, and eosinophilic bronchitis. In general, leukocytosis is rarely caused by an eosinophilia only.

The stress-induced release of endogenous corticosteroids or the administration of exogenous corticosteroids results in an eosinopenia. Corticosteroids and ACTH neutralize histamine and thus reduce stimulation for bone marrow production. Overwhelming release of histamine can negate the effects of systemic stress and produce lymphopenia, neutrophilia, and eosinophilia. Administration of ACTH or prednisolone produces eosinopenia for 4 to 8 hours and blood values return to normal in 24 hours after one dose of prednisolone.[1] Hyperadrenocorticism commonly causes an eosinopenia. An animal may remain eosinopenic for one week after prolonged corticosteroid therapy is discontinued. Diseases, intoxications, and trauma result in systemic stress-induced eosinopenia.

Basocytophilia

Basocytophilia seldom occurs and little is known of its function. It can appear along with dirofilariasis, chronic respiratory disease, and possibly with hyperadrenocorticism. The number of basophils in the peripheral blood is inversely related to the number of mast cells in the tissue. The lysosomes of basophils are similar to the lysosomes of mast cells in that they contain histamine and heparin.

Lymphocytosis

Lymphocytosis occurs in dogs when blood values exceed 4800 cells/μl, and in cats when they exceed 7000 cells/μl.[1] Absolute values should be used when dealing with lymphocytes. Young kittens and puppies have higher blood values than do adults.

Pathologic lymphocytosis occurs with lymphocytic leukemia, adrenal insufficiency, and prolonged antigenic stimulation (chronic infection, hypersensitivities, and autoimmune diseases). The degree of stress associated with these diseases has a corresponding effect on the lymphocyte value.

Atypical lymphocytes are found in cases of antigenic stimulation. This is the usual cause of benign morphologic change in lymphocytes. These lymphocytes are larger, and may have an eccentric nucleus with nucleoli and an intense basophilic cytoplasm.

Lymphopenia

Lymphopenia results when blood lymphocyte values are less than 1000/μl in dogs and 1500/μl in cats.[2]

Tissue redistribution associated with administration of corticosteroids, hyperadrenocorticism, and systemic stress can cause a reduction in the number of circulating lymphocytes. Extravasation from chylothorax and chronic enteric disease reduces the availability. Infectious agents (viral, bacterial, rickettsial, protozoal) all can reduce the lymphocyte count.

Monocytosis

Absolute monocytosis occurs with blood levels that exceed 1350/μl in dogs and 850/μl in cats.[1] Monocytosis often occurs with chronic infections. Suppuration, necrosis, malignancies, and hemorrhage into tissues cause monocytes to migrate from the blood to be transformed into tissue macrophages. Monocytes usually are seen later in an inflammatory reaction than are neutrophils. This probably occurs because of the longer half-life of monocytes. Chronic abscesses, anemias, arthritis, and cystitis can cause monocytosis. Corticosteroids and systemic stress in dogs and occasionally in cats can induce monocytosis.

REFERENCES

1. Ettinger, S.J.: *Textbook of Veterinary Internal Medicine*, vol. 2. W.B. Saunders, Philadelphia, Pa., 1975.
2. Benjamin, M.M.: *Outline of Veterinary Clinical Pathology*, 3rd ed. The Iowa State University Press, Ames, Iowa, 1978.
3. Schalm, O.W. *et al*: *Veterinary Hematology*, 3rd ed. Lea & Febiger, Philadelphia, Pa., 1975.

CHAPTER 11

Examination of the bone marrow

THE BONE MARROW is the principal site of hemopoiesis in normal adult animals. The primary function of bone marrow is the production and maturation of erythrocytes, granulocytes, monocytes, and platelets. Production of lymphocytes in the bone marrow is limited, the main source of circulating lymphocytes being the spleen and peripheral lymphatic tissue.

Evaluation of bone marrow is indicated in situations where there is a problem in the hemopoietic system that cannot adequately be diagnosed by examination of the peripheral blood. The bone marrow evaluation in conjunction with evaluation of the peripheral blood smear, can be used to diagnose leukemias, determine abnormalities of blood-cell types, determine the cause of and help classify anemias, investigate body stores of iron, confirm neoplasia, and demonstrate the presence of certain pathogenic organisms (*e.g. Histoplasma, Ehrlichia, Toxoplasma*). The bone marrow examination should be performed on cases of nonregenerative anemias, pancytopenias, neutropenias, thrombocytopenias, and myeloproliferative disorders.

Normal bone marrow is composed of vascular sinuses supported by mesenchymal cells whose contents are part of the circulating blood. Hemopoiesis takes place in the vascular sinuses. The active part of the bone marrow is the red marrow; the inactive part is the yellow marrow. In adults, red marrow is found mostly in the flat bones, short bones, and the ends of the long bones. Sites normally containing red marrow throughout an animal's life are the ribs, sternum, femur, and iliac crest.

The most common sites for aspiration of bone marrow are the trochanteric fossa of the femur in cats and the greater iliac crest in dogs. If a core biopsy specimen is needed, the greater iliac crest is the preferred site in both species.

Equipment

The needle used for aspiration of bone marrow should be of strong steel, have a short-beveled point, and have a large hub that can easily be grasped. Our preference is the University of Illinois sternal biopsy needle (V. Mueller Co.) or the Rosenthal needle for bone marrow biopsies (Becton-Dickinson). These needles can be obtained in 16- or 18-gauge widths and 1.0- or 1.5-inch lengths. Each needle contains a stylet that will fill the bore of the needle and keep bone particles from obstructing the lumen when the needle is inserted into the marrow. The stylet is removed when aspiration is performed. The needle is relatively inexpensive, durable, and easily cleaned and maintained. The large hub of the Rosenthal needle facilitates its manipulation through the dense cortical bone. The University of Illinois needle has a guard that prevents it from penetrating too deeply, but because the needle is short, its use is limited to superficial bone marrow sites.

A glass syringe should be used for aspiration of the bone marrow; however, a disposable plastic syringe with good suction is acceptable. Because of the short coagulation time of marrow, the interior of the syringe should be coated with a liquid anticoagulant, preferably EDTA. This is easily accomplished by drawing a drop of EDTA solution into the barrel of the syringe and moving the plunger to allow the EDTA to coat the syringe. Enough EDTA is

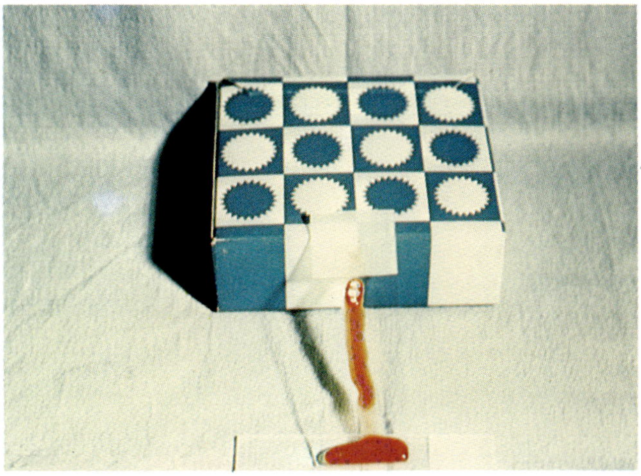

Figure 1—Marrow is expelled from the syringe onto an inclined glass slide and peripheral blood, which might contaminate the smear, is allowed to run off.

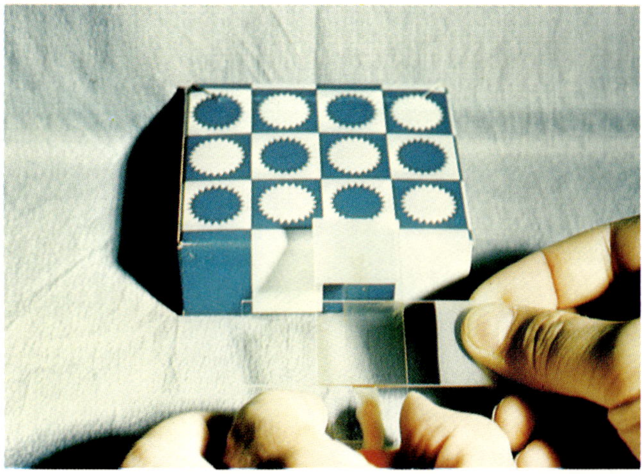

Figure 2—To make the bone marrow smear, a clean glass slide is drawn perpendicularly across the inclined slide containing bone marrow aspirate.

obtained by this method to prevent the marrow from coagulating.

Other equipment needed for aspiration of bone marrow includes a scalpel, local anesthetic agent, glass slides, and materials for surgical preparation.

Procedure

When bone marrow is aspirated from the iliac crest, the animal should be standing or on its side with the hind legs extended. For aspirations of bone marrow from the trochanteric fossa, the animal is in lateral recumbency. The area over the dorsal aspect of the iliac crest or the area over the greater trochanter is clipped and prepared for aseptic surgery. One-half to 2 ml of a local anesthetic is injected beneath the skin and into and around the periosteum. If necessary, the animal can be anesthetized with a general anesthetic. Aspiration of bone marrow causes slight discomfort. The patient will feel some pain because of the nervous tissue in the marrow.

A small stab incision is made through the skin over the site chosen for the aspiration. The needle, with stylet in place, is inserted and advanced to the center of the widest part of the iliac crest or trochanteric fossa. With the skin held taut, the needle is positioned at a right angle to the bone and gently but firmly rotated until it penetrates the cortex and is implanted in the marrow cavity. Once in place, the needle remains there unsupported.

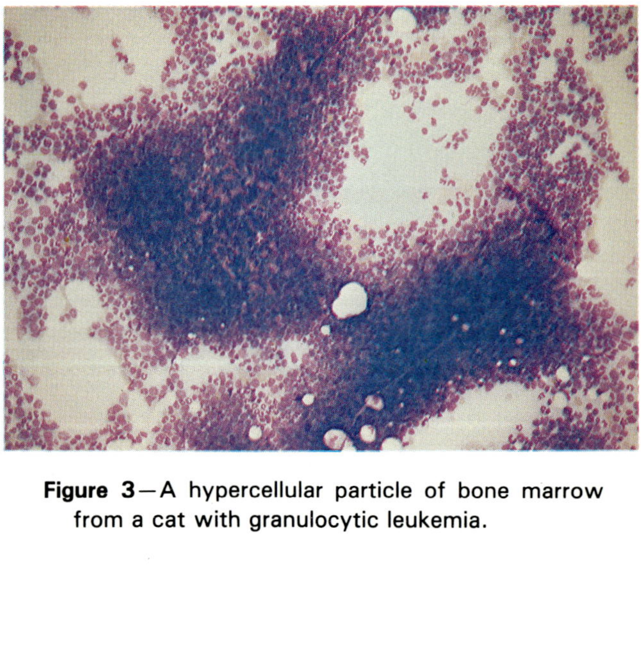

Figure 3—A hypercellular particle of bone marrow from a cat with granulocytic leukemia.

The stylet is then removed from the needle and a 20-cc syringe is locked onto the needle. Marrow is aspirated by quickly pulling the plunger back as far as possible to create a sudden negative pressure. To facilitate aspiration of the marrow, intermittent application of suction might be needed. This is done to dislodge solid marrow tissue in the needle. Aspiration should cease as soon as a few drops of marrow appear in the syringe. Too much aspiration from prolonged suction will cause the bone marrow to become diluted with peripheral blood, especially in an anemic animal.

The syringe and needle are removed from the animal and the marrow is expelled from the syringe onto a vertically inclined glass slide (*Figure 1*). This allows blood which might contaminate the speci-

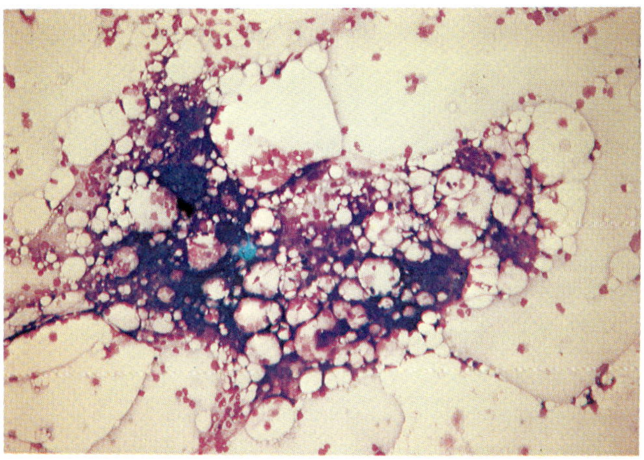

Figure 4—A hypocellular particle of bone marrow from a kitten with panleukopenia.

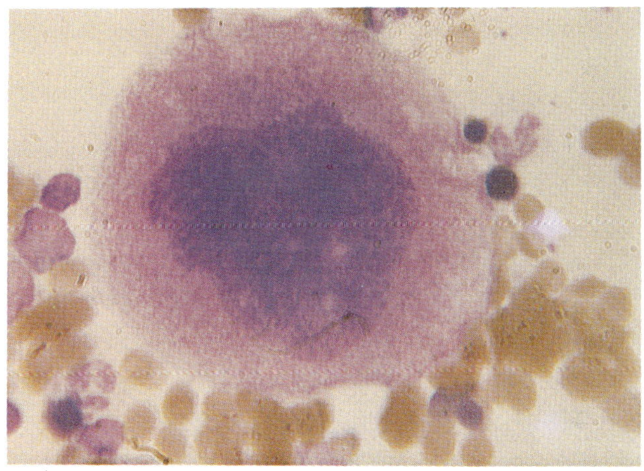

Figure 5—A megakaryocyte, the largest cell in normal bone marrow and precursor of thrombocytes.

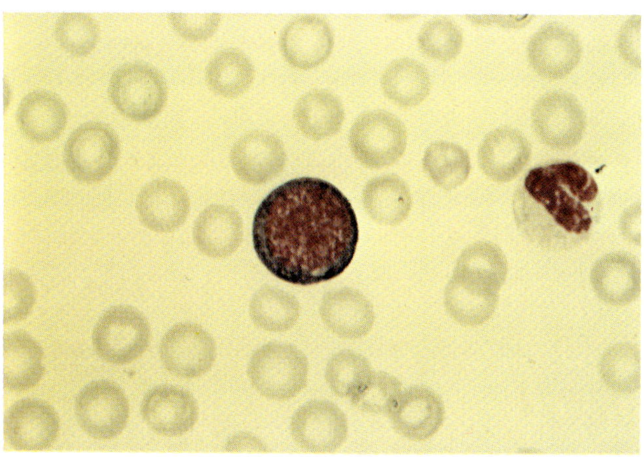

Figure 6—A prorubricyte, precursor of erythrocytes.

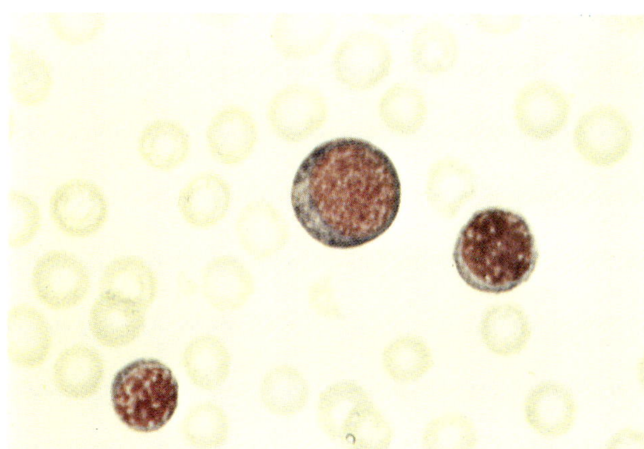

Figure 7—Three rubricytes in various stages of maturation. The largest is the most immature.

men, to run off the slide and leaves spicules of marrow on the surface of the slide. Another clean glass slide is drawn perpendicularly across this slide, to spread out the marrow (*Figure 2*). The slide is then rapidly air-dried.

The slide can be stained by the same methods used to stain a peripheral blood smear.[1] Other special stains can be used (*e.g.* the presence of iron granules can be demonstrated using Prussian blue stain, and immature granulocytes can be differentiated from lymphocytes using a peroxidase stain). Procedures for using these stains can be found in standard hematology texts.

Examination

Fortunately, a detailed examination and identification of each cell type of both the erythrocytic series and leukocytic series is not usually required. A visual impression of the overall bone-marrow response, estimation of the myeloid-erythroid ratio, and a knowledge of the status of the patient's peripheral blood usually provide the data needed for effective evaluation of the hemopoietic system.

TABLE 1—Interpretation of the M:E ratio*

1. Normal M:E ratio
   a. Normal marrow
   b. Myelosclerosis
   c. Aplastic anemias
2. Increased M:E ratio
   a. Leukocytosis
   b. Leukomoid response
   c. Granulocytic leukemia
   d. Lymphosarcoma
   e. Chronic interstitial nephritis
   f. Erythroid hypoplasia
3. Decreased M:E ratio
   a. Decrease in the myeloid cells
   b. Erythroid hyperplasia
      1) Blood loss
      2) Hemolysis
      3) Iron deficiencies
      4) Lead poisonings
      5) Polycythemia vera
      6) Cirrhosis of the liver
      7) Deficiencies in B_{12} / folic acid
      8) Congenital porphyria in cattle
      9) Erythremic myelosis

* Taken in part from: Duncan, J.R.; Prasse, K.W.: *Veterinary Laboratory Medicine, Clinical Pathology.* Iowa State Univ. Press, Ames, Iowa, 1977.

If a systematic approach is used to study the smear, detailed cytology of bone marrow is not needed to gain a useful general impression of the patient's bone-marrow response.

First, to determine the cellularity of the stained smear it should be placed on the microscope and observed under low-power magnification. Figure 3 is a photomicrograph of a bone-marrow smear showing *hyper*cellularity; Figure 4 is a photomicrograph of a smear showing *hypo*cellularity. The appearance of a normal smear is somewhere between these extremes. While the microscope is on low-power magnification, the largest cells of the bone marrow, the megakaryocytes, should be observed. The megakaryocyte (*Figure 5*) is a large, multinucleated cell; its cytoplasmic fragments are the source of blood platelets.

A peripheral thrombocytopenia without the presence of megakaryocytes in the bone marrow means the prognosis is poor and usually indicates viral destruction of the stem cell. A peripheral thrombocytopenia with the presence of megakaryocytes supports a better prognosis and usually indicates autoimmune destruction or splenic sequestration of the platelets, or both.

Next, the smear should be observed at higher magnification. If there is a general monomorphism, *i.e.* all the cells look alike, a diagnosis of neoplasia must be considered, and if possible the cell type should be identified. If a general monomorphism is not a feature, the erythrocytic and leukocytic series should be examined separately. The cells of the erythrocytic maturation series have a round nucleus and a cytoplasm that is basophilic in immature cells (*Figure 6*) and eosinophilic in mature cells. They become more eosinophilic as hemoglobin is synthetized in the cytoplasm. Figure 7 shows cells in the rubricytic stage of maturation. Ninety percent of the erythrocytic series should be at or beyond this stage of maturation in a normal animal.

The cells of the leukocytic series can be differentiated from those of the erythrocytic series by the shape of their nuclei and by cytoplasmic staining.

A detailed description of maturation and morphology of the leukocytic series has been given.[2] Eighty percent of the leukocytic series should have an indented nucleus and the cytoplasm should have granules (*i.e.* neutrophilic, eosinophilic, or basophilic granules).

Last, the myeloid-erythroid (M:E) ratio should be determined. This ratio expresses the proportion of the total number of leukocytic (myeloid) cells to the total number of nucleated erythrocytic (erythroid) cells. The ratio is determined by the formula:

$$\text{M:E} = \frac{\text{Number of myeloid cells}}{\text{Number of erythroid cells}}$$

A total of 500 nucleated cells are counted and classified as myeloid or erythroid. The normal M:E ratio should be between 0.75 and 2.0:1.0.

Interpretation of the M:E ratio depends on knowing the status of the patient's peripheral blood; *e.g.*, an M:E ratio of 5:1 (five times as many myeloid cells as erythroid cells) would mean:

1. Myeloid hyperplasia if the peripheral white blood cell (WBC) count is elevated and the packed cell volume (PCV) is normal,
2. Erythroid hypoplasia if the peripheral WBC count is normal and the PCV is decreased.

The converse is also true; a M:E ratio of 0.2 (also expressed as 1:5) could mean myeloid hypoplasia in the presence of leukopenia with a normal PCV, or erythroid hyperplasia in the presence of a normal WBC count and a regenerative anemia. The relationships of normal and altered M:E ratios to various disease states are summarized in Table 1.

*****

Note: Detailed descriptions and photomicrographs of individual cells of the erythrocytic and leukocytic series can be found in several texts on veterinary hematology. *Bone Marrow Evaluation in Veterinary Practice* (published by Ralston Purina Co.) is notable for its photomicrographs and descriptions of cellular morphology of bone marrow.

REFERENCES

1. Seybold, I.M. *et al*: The Basic Clinical Pathology Laboratory—5: Evaluation of the Blood Smear. *VM/SAC* 75(5):781-789; May 1980.
2. Wilkes, R.D. *et al*: The Clinical Pathology Laboratory—8: Evaluation of the Leukocytes: Morphology, Production, Maturation, and Function. *VM/SAC* 75(8):1233-1239; August 1980.

3 Evaluation of the urinary system

CHAPTER 12

Urinalysis:

the physical and chemical examination

THE AMOUNT OF URINE an animal produces depends on diet, fluid intake, climate, exercise, size, and weight. Accurate ranges are not available for all species but the dog's urine output ranges from 12 to 20 ml/lb/24 hours.

Urine is normally yellow to light amber, depending on the concentration of urochrome pigments, which are produced daily in relatively consistent amounts. This concentration depends on the volume of urine produced in a given period. Colorless urine may be normal or may be related to diseases that cause polyuria such as end-stage kidney disease, diabetes insipidus, pyometra, or hyperadrenocorticism. Dark, yellow-brown urine may be normal or it may relate to problems that cause high specific gravity and low urine volume, *e.g.* fever, dehydration, or acute nephritis.

Yellow-brown to greenish-yellow urine indicates an increase in biliverdin, bilirubin, or urobilin; hepatic disease is the usual cause. Red or brown urine indicates hematuria or hemoglobinuria. Brown to brownish-black urine may be indicative of hemoglobin, bile, or methemoglobin.

Urine specific gravity

The normal specific gravity of urine in the dog is 1.015 to 1.045 and in the cat is 1.020 to 1.040. A range for urine specific gravity of 1.001 to 1.060 may be normal in both the cat and dog, depending on hydration status.[1] Specific gravity is usually inversely related to urine volume. In generalized renal disease, a low specific gravity is usually found regardless of urine volume. All parameters of urinalysis should be interpreted in light of specific gravity. A specific gravity above or below the isosthenuric or fixed range (1.008 to 1.012) indicates the kidneys can actively function. Specific gravity may be within this fixed range and be normal.

Follow-up examination should be done to ascertain any pathologic change. Clinical evidence of dehydration, increased packed cell volume (PCV) and plasma proteins, and a specific gravity within the fixed range indicate that antidiuretic hormone is not being released properly (diabetes insipidus) or that the kidneys are unable to respond to antidiuretic hormone (renal diabetes insipidus or generalized kidney disease). A fixed specific gravity along with elevated blood urea nitrogen (BUN) or elevated creatinine are indicative of generalized kidney disease.

Pathologic causes of increased specific gravity include dehydration from any cause: fever, edema, burns, initial stages of acute nephritis, certain stages of diabetes mellitus, primary renal glucosuria, shock, and conditions that allow large numbers of particles to accumulate in the urine.

Pathologic causes of decreased specific gravity include chronic generalized nephritis, acute generalized nephritis, renal amyloidosis, generalized pyelonephritis, diabetes insipidus, pyometra, hyperadrenocorticism, and certain generalized diseases of the liver. The specific gravity of chronic or severe acute nephritis may become fixed. Specific gravity is usually measured with a refractometer but a urinometer can be used.

Urine protein

A semi-quantitative evaluation of urine protein can be obtained by using a reagent strip or acid precipitation test. Positive reactions on most reagent strips are measured as 1+, 2+, 3+, or 4+, which are equivalent to 30 mg, 100 mg, 300 mg, and 1000 mg protein/dl, respectively.[2] The acid precipitation tests also have a scale of 1+ through 4+.

In general, tests in which reagent strips are used tend to give false positive readings at low protein concentrations.[1] Because of this discrepancy, positive reagent strip readings should be verified by using other laboratory tests for proteinuria such as the sulfosalicylic acid turbidimetric method. This acid precipitation test also may help rule out false positive readings that can occur when urine is alkaline. As a quantitative test, the sulfosalicylic acid turbidimetric method (Bumintest® —Ames) can be used to measure total protein excretion for a 24-hour period; this is the best measurement, but semi-quantitative measurements are most commonly used.

In most cases, specific gravity and urine volume are inversely proportional, and both should be examined when estimating the amount of protein being excreted. Strenuous exercise and stress may cause nonpathologic accumulation of protein in the urine. Physiologic proteinuria is usually transient in duration. A nonpathologic increase in urine protein may also be found in newborn animals.

Pathologic proteinuria can be caused by hemorrhagic, inflammatory, and glomerular and/or tubular disease; causes of these diseases may be of renal or nonrenal origin. Renal diseases result in a greater loss of albumin than of globulins. The quantity of protein excreted by an animal does not necessarily indicate the severity of the disease.

When there is hemorrhage into the bladder, very high protein values are recorded, the urine occult blood test is positive, and erythrocytes are observed in the sediment; causes may be trauma, inflammation, or neoplasia. A complete examination of the genito-urinary tract should be performed in an effort to locate the cause of the hemorrhage.

Glomerular or tubular damage should be considered when proteinuria exists without occult blood or significant cellular sediment. Glomerular disease typically has a high proteinuria and can be differentiated from tubular damage, which routinely has lower protein values. Heavy proteinuria without hematuria or pyuria indicates renal disease, especially involving the glomeruli. It should be noted that glomerular and tubular disease can occur simultaneously. Any factor that causes increased glomerular permeability, (*e.g.* fever, cardiac disease, central nervous system disease, and shock)[2] increases proteinuria. Tubular disease that slows reabsorption by the tubules increases protein in the urine. Casts found in the sediment indicate direct kidney damage.

Specific causes of renal proteinuria include renal amyloidosis (mild to severe proteinuria), acute nephritis (moderate to heavy proteinuria with casts, red blood cells [RBC], and white blood cells [WBC] in the sediment), chronic generalized nephritis (absent to mild proteinuria), pyelonephritis (mild to moderate proteinuria, often with RBC, WBC, casts, and bacteria in the sediment), polycystic kidneys (absent to moderate proteinuria), and glomerulonephritis (mild to heavy proteinuria).

Nonrenal causes of proteinuria include chronic, passive congestion of the kidneys secondary to cardiac insufficiency, or an increase in intra-abdominal pressure from tumors or ascites. Genital tract contamination and the inflammatory exudate that usually accompanies it increase the amount of protein in the urine. Protein may also be lost into the urine because of inflammatory diseases of the bladder and urethra.

Urine glucose

Urine glucose can be detected by the glucose oxidase and copper reductase methods. If glucose levels in the blood do not exceed 180 mg/100 ml, the proximal tubules resorb all glucose from the glomerular filtrate leaving the urine free of glucose.[3]

Postprandial hyperglycemia, diabetes mellitus, exertional hyperglycemia, and certain therapeutic agents may cause glucosuria. Also, severe acute pancreatitis with hypoinsulinism may be associated with glucosuria. Primary renal glucosuria can occur without the presence of other renal disease. Urine from hematuric cats may produce false positive results for glucose on the reagent strips. Urine glucose is not a test for tubular function, and a positive reading for glucosuria rarely occurs in cases of primary renal disease without concomitant hyperglycemia.

Urine ketones

The nitroprusside reaction (using the reagent strip or tablet method) can be used to detect ketones in the urine. Ketonuria results from the accumulation of acetoacetic acid, beta-hydroxybutyric acid, and acetone in the blood. Ketonuria occurs before ketonemia. Excessive metabolism of fat and/or a deficiency in the metabolism of carbohydrates are the basic abnormalities found when ketonuria is detected. Diabetes mellitus, starvation, and excessive dietary intake of fat are common causes.

Urine bilirubin

Bilirubin should be evaluated right after the urine is collected because when exposed to light, bilirubin is oxidized to biliverdin or hydrolyzed to free bilirubin, resulting in false negatives.

Both reagent strip and tablet methods are used to detect urine bilirubin. The color of the urine may cause readings from the reagent strip to be inaccurate. The tablet method is more sensitive, and 1+ readings are not considered significant.

Bilirubinuria occurs when flow of bile is obstructed and conjugated bilirubin is regurgitated into the blood stream, or when severe hemolytic disease exists. Bilirubinuria can be observed when a concomitant rise in serum bilirubin is not present.[2] Specific gravity affects the amount of bilirubin found in the urine. Urine with high specific gravity from normal dogs may contain some bilirubin, although the renal threshold for bilirubin in the dog is low. Pathologic bilirubinuria is caused by hepatocellular disease from infectious canine hepatitis, leptospirosis, cirrhosis, neoplasia, and toxicities.

Urine occult blood

Hemoglobin and myoglobin are detected by the occult blood test. Both reagent strip and tablet methods are based on the peroxidase properties of free hemoglobin or myoglobin. Free hemoglobin or myoglobin results in a positive occult blood test, but intact erythrocytes do not, unless the concentration of RBCs exceeds 10 RBCs/high power field.

Hematuria can cause an occult blood test to be positive because hemoglobin is released after hemolysis in the urine. Red, cloudy urine is usually present without evidence of anemia or muscle disease. Hemoglobinuria is characterized by red to brown urine, absence of RBCs in the sediment, evidence of anemia, and no evidence of muscle disease. Myoglobinuria is characterized by brownish urine, a lack of RBCs in the sediment, no anemia, and clinical and laboratory evidence of muscle disease.

Urine urobilinogen

Urobilinogen is usually detected with the reagent strip, a semi-quantitative method. A fresh urine sample is required because of the quick destruction of urobilinogen. Many normal animals have no detectable urobilinogen in their urine. A positive urobilinogen test indicates a patent bile duct. Absence of urobilinogen in the presence of jaundice indicates bile obstruction. Although little correlation exists between urine urobilinogen concentration and hepatic disease, an increased concentration of urobilinogen is considered to be an indication of hemolytic diseases or diseases related to decreased hepatic mass.

Urine pH

Urine pH can be measured with a variety of reagent strips. A fresh sample of urine should be used because the pH becomes more alkaline as urine ages. Normal pH ranges from 5.5 to 7.5. Dog and cat urine is normally acidic. Diet, cystitis, acid-base balance, and therapy all affect urine pH. Cystitis frequently causes urine pH to become more alkaline. The administration of sodium lactate, sodium bicarbonate, and sodium citrate may cause urine to become more alkaline.

Acidic urine may be caused by feeding animals high protein diets, the catabolism of body proteins secondary to fever, starvation, and diabetes mellitus. Uremia and diabetes mellitus are two common causes of metabolic acidosis, resulting in acidic urine. Ammonium chloride, oral calcium chloride, sodium acid phosphate, and d,L-methionine are agents that produce a more acidic pH of the urine.

REFERENCES

1. Osborne, C.A. *et al: Canine and Feline Urology*. W.B. Saunders, Philadelphia, Pa., 1972; pp 40-55.
2. Duncan, J.R.; Prasse, K.E.: *Veterinary Laboratory Medicine, Clinical Pathology*. Iowa State University Press, Ames, Iowa, 1977.
3. Benjamin, M.M.: *Outline of Veterinary Clinical Pathology*, 3rd ed. Iowa State University Press, Ames, Iowa, 1977.

CHAPTER 13

Urinalysis: examination of urine sediment

MICROSCOPIC EXAMINATION of urine is an inexpensive, and readily available laboratory test that provides useful diagnostic and prognostic information.

Urine should be collected in clean glass or plastic containers. The first urine voided in the morning is preferred because it will be more concentrated and more likely to contain abnormal constituents than urine collected at any other time of day. The first sample of the day will be free of the immediate influence of activities such as feeding and exercise.

Urine can be collected as it is voided (spontaneous urination or manual compression), or with the aid of catheterization or cystocentesis. When voided urine is collected, the initial stream should not be used because it may contain cellular debris, bacteria, and mucus from the urethra and genital tract.

Collection of urine by catheterization should be done as aseptically, gently, and atraumatically as possible. Catheters are available in a variety of diameters and lengths. The diameter of a catheter is commonly designated in French units (abbreviated as F). Three French units equal 1 mm. Radiopaque catheters are useful when the urinary system is to be radiographed.

Collection of urine by cystocentesis is preferred when a urine bacterial culture is desired.

Urine sediment should be analyzed while the urine is fresh. If urine is allowed to stand at room temperature, bacteria will multiply and cause an increase in pH that will dissolve casts and other formed elements. If the urine cannot be examined while fresh, it can be refrigerated for up to three hours. Urine can also be preserved by adding 5 to 10 drops of 10% formalin to 10 to 20 ml of urine. Formalin will alter some chemical constituents in the urine, but will not alter formed elements.

Examination of urine sediment should be standardized so that consecutive samples may be accurately compared. A good procedure is to centrifuge 10 ml of urine for five minutes at 1500 rpm. The supernatant is then decanted, leaving 0.5 ml of sediment. The sediment is gently mixed, one drop is transferred to the end of a microscope slide, and a coverslip is added. Another drop is transferred to the other end of the slide along with a drop of new methylene blue stain. Another coverslip is added. By this method, both stained and unstained sediments from a standard amount of urine can be studied on the same slide.

Stained and unstained sediments are examined first under low-power magnification with reduced illumination (lowered condenser and partial closure of the iris diaphragm). Final identification of cells and casts is made under high-power magnification and reported as average number per high dry field (HDF). If the sediment is extremely cellular as in the case of hematuria or pyuria, the cells are identified and then recorded as too numerous to count, *e.g.* WBC tntc/ HDF.

Cells that can be found in urine sediment include epithelial cells (squamous and transitional), leukocytes, and erythrocytes.

Epithelial cells

Squamous epithelial cells (*Figure 1*) are large, with irregular angular margins and very small nuclei. These cells are normal in urine sediment. They arise by desquamation from the vagina or prepuce. More of these cells are seen when the urine sample is obtained by traumatic catheterization, or when

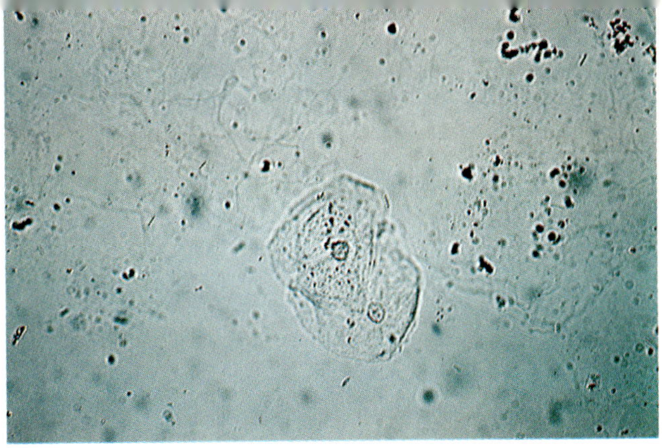

Figure 1—Squamous epithelial cells.

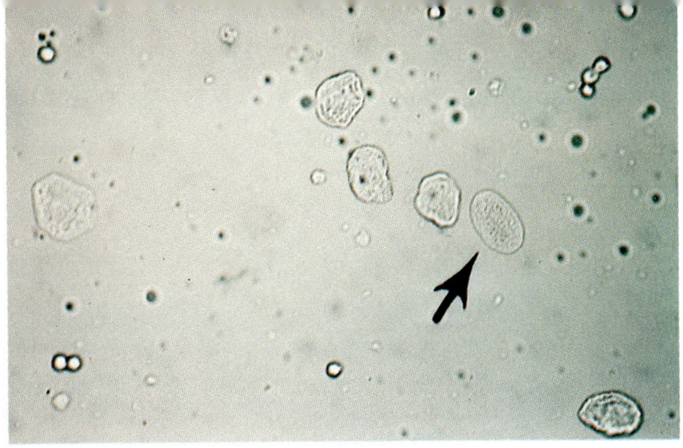

Figure 2—Transitional epithelial cells.

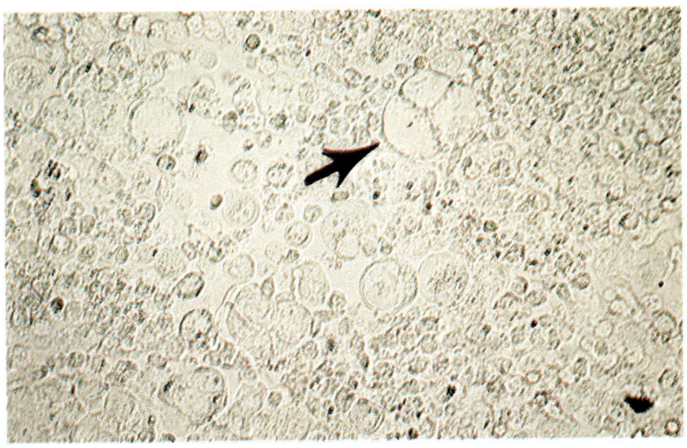

Figure 3—Neoplastic transitional epithelial cells.

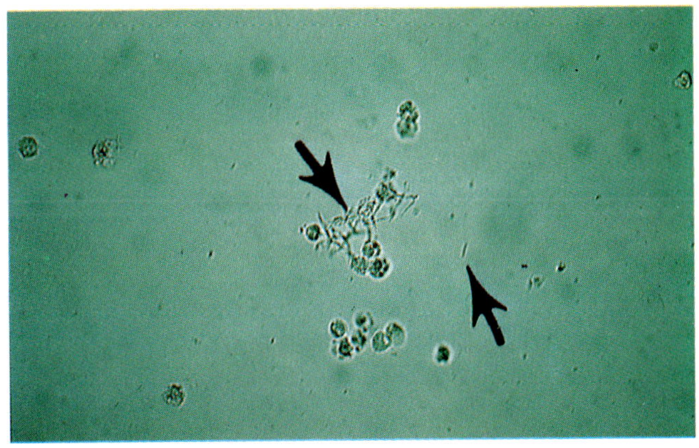

Figure 4—Leukocytes; bacteria.

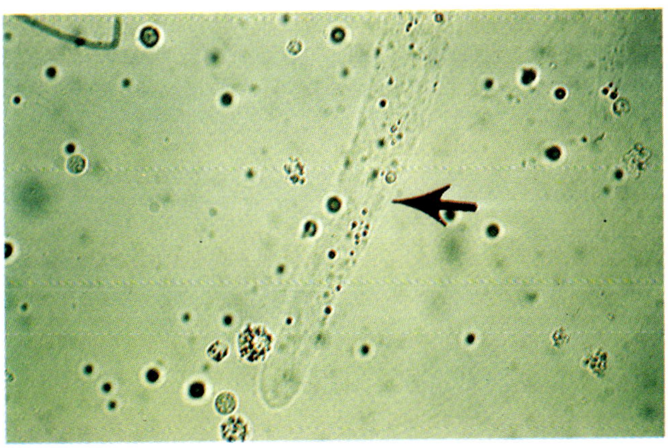

Figure 5—Hyaline cast.

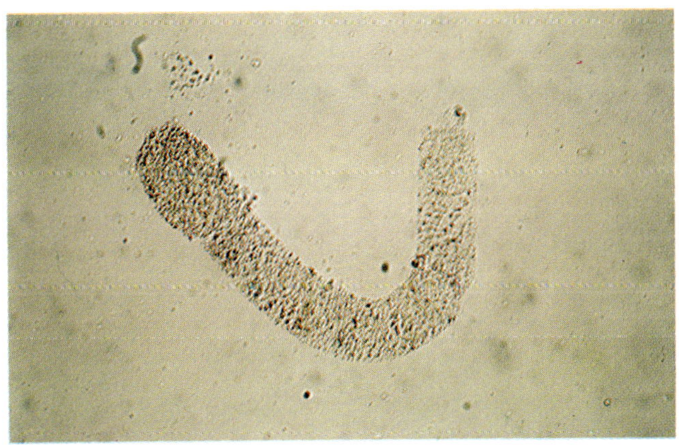

Figure 6—Granular cast.

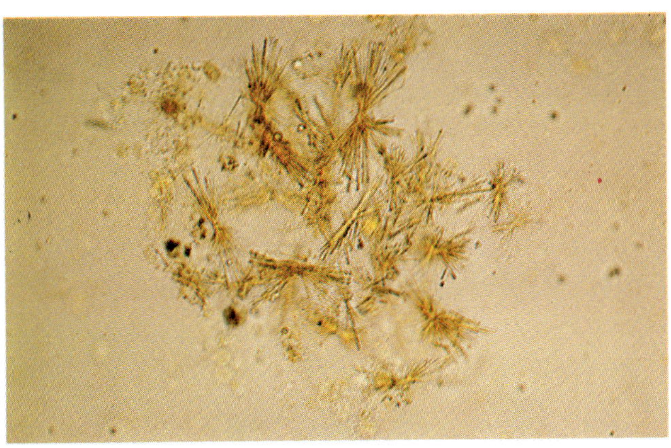

Figure 7—Tyrosine crystals.

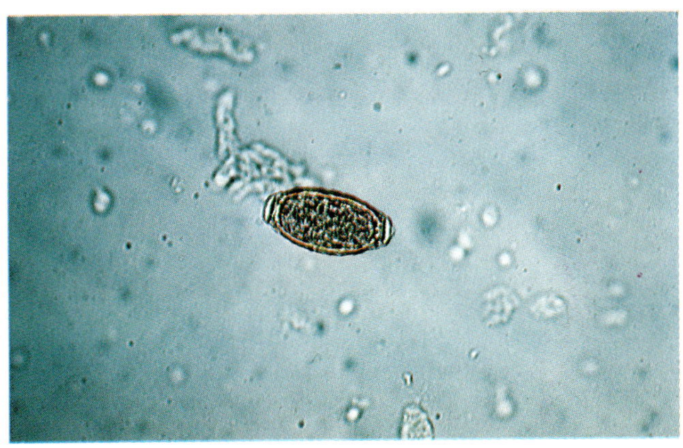

Figure 8—*Capillaria plica* eggs.

the first stream of urine from a voided sample is used in the urinalysis.

Transitional epithelial cells (*Figure 2*) usually arise from the urinary bladder or urethra but can come from the renal pelvis or ureters. Such cells are smaller than squamous epithelial cells and are usually oval. Transitional epithelial cells are only of diagnostic importance if they are neoplastic (*Figure 3*). Transitional epithelial cells that are neoplastic vary in size, have very large nuclei with prominent nucleoli, and often occur in tightly adhered clumps.

Leukocytes

Leukocytes are round and granular. They are larger than erythrocytes but smaller than epithelial cells. Leukocytes can easily be recognized on the stained portion of the slide because the nuclei prominently take new methylene blue stain. Observation of more than five leukocytes/ HDF indicates inflammation of the urogenital tract. High numbers of leukocytes, in the presence of bacteria (*Figure 4*) and absence of casts, is characteristic of cystitis and/or urethritis.

Erythrocytes

Erythrocytes are found in small numbers in normal urine sediment, especially when the sample is obtained by manual compression or catheterization. Observation of more than 5 erythrocytes/ HDF usually indicates hematuria. Erythrocytes may lyse and not be microscopically visible in dilute urine (specific gravity less than 1.010).

Casts

Casts are elongated structures formed in the kidneys from plasma protein and/or renal tubular mucoprotein. Casts are formed in the distal tubules where the urine is more acidic and has a higher osmolarity. The number of casts in urine sediment is not a direct indication of the severity of renal disease. For example, few casts may be present in sediment from patients with severe chronic nephritis and few-to-many casts may be seen in sediment from patients with acute nephropathies. All casts are formed from a protein matrix but can be differentiated by additional components from the renal tissue that combine with this protein matrix.

Hyaline casts (*Figure 5*) are colorless, homogenous casts composed of pure protein with no tubular desquamate. Hyaline casts indicate mild-to-moderate glomerular leakage of protein.

Granular casts (*Figure 6*) are derived from protein impregnated with degenerate fragments of epithelial cells from the renal tubules. This is the most common type of cast found in animals. The presence of such casts indicates damage to the renal tubules.

Cellular casts occur when recognizable (nondegenerate) cells combine with a protein matrix. They are named according to the cell type found in the cast. Leukocytic casts are cellular, contain leukocytes, and indicate pyelonephritis. Erythrocytic casts are cellular, contain erythrocytes, and indicate renal hemorrhage. Epithelial casts are cellular, contain epithelial cells from renal tubules, and indicate damage to renal tubules.

Fatty casts contain fat globules from degenerating tubular epithelial cells. Fatty casts are often seen in cats because of the high lipid content of the epithelium in the feline renal tubule.

Crystals are often found in urine sediment. They are seldom clinically significant, so identification is usually not worthwhile. Crystals that are clinically significant are ammonium biurate and tyrosine (*Figure 7*), which are seen in cases of hepatic damage. Cysteine crystals are seen in cases of congenital cystinuria. Charts for identification of crystals can be found in clinical pathology texts.

Miscellaneous structures also found in urine sediment include: fat, sperm, and contaminant fungal hyphae. Parasitic ova, especially *Capillaria plica* eggs (*Figure 8*) are found occasionally.

CHAPTER 14

Evaluation of renal function—1:
blood urea nitrogen and creatinine determinations

SUCCESSFUL DIAGNOSIS, prognosis, and treatment of animals with renal disease require the use and understanding of several laboratory procedures. Blood urea nitrogen (BUN) values, creatinine values, urinalysis, urine concentration test, and the phenolsulfonphthalein (PSP) excretion test are commonly used in evaluating renal disease.

In this chapter, we present methods used to determine and interpret BUN and serum creatinine values. Serum levels of nonprotein nitrogen substances, especially urea and creatinine, are often used as indicators of renal function.

Blood urea nitrogen (BUN)

Urea is produced in the liver from catabolized protein. It is excreted through glomerular filtration in the kidneys. Urea is a small molecule (MW = 60). Because urea passively diffuses across the glomerular membrane, BUN is a gross indicator of the rate of glomerular filtration. Normal BUN levels for dogs and cats range from 10 mg/dl to 30 mg/dl. The range may vary slightly among laboratories.

Elevated BUN levels occur when the rate of urea production increases or when the rate of excretion decreases. High-protein diets may cause the BUN level to become mildly elevated (35 to 45 mg/dl). To determine whether diet is the cause of an elevated BUN level, the animal should be fasted for 12 to 18 hours before the BUN measurement is repeated. A mild to moderate elevation of the BUN level in an anorexic animal is more severe than the same elevation in an animal on a high-protein diet.

Any factor that increases the catabolism of protein can cause an elevated BUN level. Exogenous causes of increased catabolism of protein include corticosteroids, thyroid hormones, and tetracyclines. Fever, infection, trauma, and gastrointestinal hemorrhage are endogenous causes of increased catabolism of protein. Primary renal disease will cause a reduced rate of urea excretion. But 75% of the functional nephrons must be lost before the BUN level becomes significantly elevated. As nephrons in the kidney are destroyed, remaining functional nephrons undergo compensatory hypertrophy. For this reason, the BUN test is not a reliable indicator of renal disease in the early stages.

A reduced rate of urea excretion is also seen with any condition that reduces the flow of blood to the kidneys. Subsequently, the rate of glomerular filtration is decreased. Cardiovascular diseases, shock, Addison's disease, and dehydration can cause a decrease in renal arterial perfusion, thereby resulting in elevated levels of both BUN and creatinine. Because the kidneys are usually normal, elevation of BUN and creatinine levels from these causes is referred to as prerenal azotemia. When elevated because of *prerenal azotemia*, BUN levels are usually less than 100 mg/dl. In these conditions the kidney should be able to concentrate urine to a specific gravity of 1.030 or greater.

A reduced rate of urea excretion also occurs with obstructive uropathies and/or rupture of a urinary segment. An elevation of the BUN or creatinine level from one of these causes is referred to as *postrenal azotemia*. Oliguria and anuria are often present. During physical and radiographic examinations the cause of the uropathy is usually found. If the obstruction and/or rupture is corrected, BUN and creatinine levels return to normal in a few days.

Creatinine

Creatine and phosphocreatinine are converted to creatinine in the muscles. Creatinine is not used by the body and is therefore excreted in the urine. In normal animals, the production and excretion of creatinine remains constant from day to day. Creatinine is freely filtered by the glomerulus. Any factors that decrease the rate of glomerular filtration cause an increase in the level of serum creatinine.

The normal creatinine level for dogs and cats ranges from 1 to 2 mg/dl. Diet and catabolic factors do not significantly affect creatinine levels. Therefore, as an indicator of renal disease, the creatinine level is more accurate than the BUN level.

In primary renal failure, abnormal creatinine values are not seen until 70% to 75% of the nephrons are nonfunctional. In our experience, creatinine concentration is a better test than BUN on which to base the prognosis in cases of primary polyuric renal failure. The prognosis is poor for animals with creatinine levels of 5 mg/dl or more. The prognosis is grave for animals with creatinine levels of 10 mg/dl or more.

Single determinations of BUN and creatinine concentrations usually will not give reliable information as to the degree of renal disease. Serial determinations of creatinine and/or BUN values in association with serial determinations of urine specific gravity can provide reliable diagnostic and prognostic information. After water deprivation, or in dehydrated animals, persistent azotemia accompanied by a urine specific gravity between 1.008 and 1.012 indicates severe renal disease. Uremia with a urine specific gravity greater than 1.030 is often a favorable sign. This indicates a sufficient number of functional nephrons to concentrate urine and that the uremia may be of prerenal origin.

Methods

Many techniques are available for determining BUN and creatinine concentrations. The most common methods involve a colorimeter or spectrophotometer and prepackaged reagent kits. These devices are reasonably accurate and provide reproducible results. The tests permit quick in-hospital determination of BUN and creatinine levels.

For practitioners without these instruments and with no available laboratory, there are several screening tests for the determination of BUN. The most common screening test is Azostix® (Ames). In this test, a strip impregnated with urease undergoes a change in color proportional to the amount of urea present in one drop of venous or capillary blood. Exactly one minute is allowed for the reaction. There are color blocks of standards for 10, 20, 30, and 50 mg/dl. This screening test provides only semi-quantitative estimates. It is not intended to replace more precise determinations.

The Bun-O-Graph® (Haver-Lockhart) and Urograph® (Warner-Chilcott) are also used to estimate BUN. They use paper chromatography and do not require colorimeters or spectrophotometers.

Measuring creatinine concentration is not as simple as measuring BUN, but colorimetric and spectrophotometric procedures are available. There are no reliable dipstick screening procedures to measure creatinine concentration.

CHAPTER 15

Renal function—2:
water-deprivation response test, exogenous antidiuretic hormone response test, and phenolsulfonphthalein-excretion test

SEVERAL TESTS can be used to evaluate renal function when routine tests such as urine specific gravity (including a complete urinalysis), blood urea nitrogen (BUN), and serum creatinine are not diagnostic. If results of these tests are inconclusive, more in-depth analysis can be gained from studies to evaluate the kidney's ability to excrete certain dyes, renal clearance tests, water deprivation response tests, and exogenous antidiuretic hormone (ADH) response tests. Renal biopsy may also be considered when a definitive diagnosis is required. However, no single test can be used for complete evaluation of renal function.

Water-deprivation response test

Patients suspected of having renal disease and having urine specific gravity values of less than 1.020 should be considered candidates for the water-deprivation test. Usually, these patients are presented with polyuria and urine specific gravity values within the normal range. Dehydrated animals are already being stimulated to produce endogenous ADH and should not be subjected to a water-deprivation test. Also, an animal with azotemia and polyuria should not be deprived of water because this may exacerbate the disease.

When water intake is restricted, ADH secretion from the posterior pituitary gland is stimulated. By increasing the distal tubular cells' permeability to water, ADH increases fluid resorption by the distal tubules and collecting ducts. A normal animal responds by excreting urine with an increased specific gravity value, high osmolarity, and low volume.

In severely polyuric animals it is important to prevent extreme dehydration during water deprivation. At the beginning of the test, urine specific gravity values and the body weight are measured. To prevent extreme dehydration, the test is stopped if the animal loses more than 7% of the body weight. Food with a low moisture content can be fed to the animal during the test.

The animal is deprived of water until its ability to concentrate urine has been determined. This usually takes between 24 and 36 hours. To prevent mixing of dilute and concentrated urine, the bladder should be emptied 12 hours after the test is begun. Urine is then collected at random intervals, and the specific gravity is measured. If the specific gravity exceeds 1.030 for dogs or 1.035 for cats, the test should be stopped. This indicates that the kidneys have the ability to concentrate urine. The test is continued until the animal loses 7% of the body weight, the specific gravity value remains below 1.030, or the animal becomes azotemic.

Failure of an animal to concentrate its urine indicates generalized renal disease, impaired production or release of ADH (diabetes insipidus [specific gravity of 1.001 to 1.006]), or impaired tubular response to ADH (renal diabetes insipidus).

Exogenous ADH response test (Table 1)

As with water deprivation, exogenous administration of ADH is used to evaluate the kidney's ability to concentrate urine. Exogenous ADH (vasopressin) is preferred for animals that are debilitated, animals in which overt renal disease may occur from water deprivation, and animals in which water deprivation was unsuccessful in producing concentrated urine. If water deprivation fails to increase the specific gravity and exogenous ADH increases the specific gravity, diabetes insipidus is diagnosed.

Two forms of ADH are available. The shorter acting aqueous form is preferred over repositol ADH. An exact dosage schedule or procedure for giving exogenous ADH has not been developed.

During the test, food should be withheld and water given *ad libitum*. The aqueous form of ADH is freshly prepared and slowly given intravenously. It is usually given for 90 minutes in 25 to 50 ml of 5% dextrose in water. The dosage is 3 to 5 mU/lb.[1]

Thirty minutes after the infusion is begun, the bladder should be emptied by catheterization. Urine is collected and specific gravity is recorded at 30, 60, 90, 120, and 180 minutes. The test can be stopped when the specific gravity exceeds 1.030.

The ADH-response test can also be performed with vasopressin in oil (Pitressin® tannate in oil—Parke-Davis). Food and water are withheld during this test. Vasopressin is injected intramuscularly at a dose of 2 to 5 units.[1]

To prevent mixing of dilute and concentrated urine, the bladder is emptied three to six hours after vasopressin is injected. Urine is collected and specific gravity recorded at 3, 6, and 9 hours.

In response to administration of exogenous ADH, a normal animal should excrete urine with a specific gravity considerably higher than the glomerular filtrate. The specific gravity should be greater than 1.030. If the specific gravity continues to be less than 1.020, the renal tubules are being impaired so that they cannot concentrate urine. This, impairment may be caused by generalized kidney disease or inability of the tubules to respond to ADH stimulation (renal diabetes insipidus).

Phenolsulfonphthalein (PSP) excretion test (Table 2)

Phenolsulfonphthalein (PSP) dye is also used to evaluate renal function. Unlike BUN and creatinine tests, a PSP excretion test can be used to detect acute renal disease. In chronic renal disease it can provide a good evaluation of functional tubular tissue. A PSP excretion test is indicated when primary kidney disease is suspected. It can also be used to evaluate generalized kidney disease when the specific gravity is fixed.

After it is injected into a vein, PSP dye attaches to plasma proteins and is excreted in the urine. The proximal renal tubules secrete 90% to 95% of PSP dye; 10% is filtered by the glomerulus, and a small amount is removed by the liver.

At the beginning of the PSP excretion test, the bladder is emptied. The bladder need not be completely empty because the total quantity of dye, not urine volume, is being measured. Six milligrams (2 ml) of the PSP is injected intravenously and the time is recorded. If the patient has not been catheterized, a catheter is inserted with the tip just beyond the neck of the bladder. All urine is collected.

The catheterization and aspiration of urine begins about 10 minutes after injection of dye and should be completed precisely 20 minutes after the injection. During this time, the bladder can be rinsed three to four times with 10 to 15 ml of sterile physiological saline solution. Fluid and urine are placed in the same flask. Repeatedly injecting 10 to 15 ml of air into the bladder after the final rinse improves dye collection.

After the urine is collected, it is diluted to 400 ml with water in a 1-liter flask. Ten milliliters of 10% sodium hydroxide is added and the solution is mixed thoroughly. If the mixture turns deep pink, water is added to make a total of 1000 ml. If the mixture is light pink, water is added to bring the total to 500 ml, and the results are divided by two. If it is turbid, the mixture should be filtered.

Another dosage regimen is 100 mg PSP/m^2 of body surface. This may be a better indication of tubular function.[2]

Generally, two methods are used to determine the quantity of dye excreted: the spectrophotome-

TABLE 1—Exogenous ADH Response Test

Exogenous Aqueous ADH Response Test

1. Withhold food during the test.
2. Prepare the aqueous ADH (vasopressin).
3. Add 2 to 5 mU/lb body weight to 25 to 50 ml 5% dextrose in water and slowly infuse intravenously.
4. Thirty minutes after injection, catheterize and empty the bladder.
5. Collect urine and record specific gravity at 30, 60, 90, 120, and 180 minutes.

Exogenous ADH in Oil Response Test

1. Intramuscularly inject 3 to 5 units of vasopressin tannate in oil.
2. Withhold all food and water during test.
3. Remove all urine from bladder three hours after injection.
4. Collect urine and record specific gravity at 3, 6, and 9 hours.

TABLE 2—Phenolsulfonphthalein (PSP) Excretion Test

1. Empty bladder by catheterization or micturition.
2. Inject 6 mg PSP dye intravenously and note time.
3. Starting at about 10 minutes after injection, collect urine and place in a flask.
4. Rinse bladder three to four times with sterile saline solution.
5. Complete urine collection at exactly 20 minutes after injection.

ter and the PSP comparator block. A colorimeter and a Unitest® (Bio-Dynamics) method have been described.[3]

When a spectrophotometer is used, a small amount of urine-dye mix is placed in a curvette. After the wavelength is set at 550 mμ, the optical density is determined.

The color of the unknown sample can be compared to color standards of a comparator block. The series of standards can be prepared as follows:

50%—Add 0.5 ml of 6 mg/ml PSP to alkalinizing sodium hydroxide and dilute with water to 500 ml.

40%—Add 8 ml of 50% standard to 2 ml water.

30%—Add 6 ml of 50% standard to 4 ml water.

20%—Add 4 ml of 50% standard to 6 ml water.

10%—Add 2 ml of 50% standard to 8 ml water.

Hemoglobin, bilirubin, and sulfobromophthalein dye will interfere with the results of this test.

The average normal excretion in 20 minutes is 43.8% (range 26-64%).[2] Young animals usually excrete 50% or more, whereas diseased animals rarely excrete more than 35%. In acute renal failure 0 to 5% PSP may be excreted. This is not enough to affect the color of the urine. Animals with chronic compensated nephritis excrete 10 to 25% of the dye, and animals with uncompensated chronic nephritis excrete 5 to 15%.[4]

An abnormal decrease in PSP excretion can be due to poor perfusion from generalized renal disease, congestive heart failure, dehydration, or hypoadrenocorticism. Generalized tubular destruction from toxins, heavy metals, or poisons may increase PSP retention. Errors in collection may cause incorrectly low values.

Other tests are available for the quantitative evaluation of kidney function. Glomerular filtration rate and renal clearance tests can give valuable information, but because of the cost and time required, routine use of these tests is prohibitive. However, when quantitative measurements of renal function are needed or acute renal failure is suspected, these tests should be considered.

REFERENCES

1. Ettinger, S.J.: *Textbook of Veterinary Internal Medicine.* W.B. Saunders, Philadelphia, Pa., 1975; pp 1477-1484.
2. Osborne, C.A. *et al: Canine and Feline Urology.* W.B. Saunders, Philadelphia, Pa., 1972; p 71.
3. Morgan, H.C.: *Practitioner's Laboratory.* Veterinary Medicine Publishing Co., Bonner Springs, Kan., 1971; pp 103-108.
4. Coles, E.H.: *Veterinary Clinical Pathology.* 2nd ed. W.B. Saunders, Philadelphia, Pa., 1974; pp 265-268.

CHAPTER 16

Renal function—3:
evaluation, treatment, and management of patients with chronic primary renal failure

CHRONIC PRIMARY renal failure, caused by a loss of more than 75% of functional renal mass, results in uremia. Progressive loss of functional renal mass induces surviving nephrons to undergo compensatory hypertrophy. To keep the animal's metabolism balanced, these nephrons increase in both size and metabolic activity. When the compensated renal mass is reduced to less than 20% of normal, clinical signs of uremia become evident.

Clinical signs most commonly seen in patients with uremia include: polydipsia, polyuria, anorexia, nausea, vomiting, anemia, osteodystrophy, metabolic acidosis, neurologic disturbances (*e.g.* lethargy, neuromuscular twitches, coma, convulsions), and hyperglycemia. The toxins of uremia cause gastrointestinal ulcerations and other gastrointestinal signs. Anemia is a result of diminished production of erythrocytes, shortened life span for erythrocytes, and gastrointestinal hemorrhage.

Abnormal metabolism of calcium and phosphorus leads to hypocalcemia and hyperphosphatemia. These conditions cause a hyperparathyroidism, which eventually results in osteodystrophy. Hypocalcemia occurs when the kidneys fail to synthesize 1,25 hydroxycholecalciferol (active vitamin D). Hyperphosphatemia occurs when the decreased glomerular filtration rate causes a reduced clearance of phosphate by the kidneys. The normal level of inorganic phosphorus in dogs and cats ranges from 3.0 to 4.5 mg/dl.

Metabolic acidosis is seen during the later stages of chronic progressive renal failure. It results from failure of the kidney to excrete acid (hydrogen ions and ammonium ions) and/or impaired ability of the renal tubules to resorb bicarbonate ions filtered by the glomerulus.

Neurologic disturbances, also seen during the later stages of renal failure, are characterized by lethargy, neuromuscular twitches, coma, and convulsions. The pathophysiologic cause of these disturbances is incompletely understood but is thought to be attributable in part to the toxins of uremia such as: urea, creatinine, and especially quanidine and methylquanidine. Other pathophysiologic explanations for the neurologic signs include excessive calcium deposits in the brain and depressed central nervous system utilization of adenosine triphosphate.

Carbohydrate intolerance characterized by persistent hyperglycemia is often seen in uremic animals. Insulin levels in the plasma are usually normal or elevated in these animals because the kidneys normally biodegrade and eliminate two-thirds of the insulin irreversibly lost from circulation. In patients with renal failure, biodegradation and renal clearance of insulin are impaired. Hyperglycemia in the presence of elevated insulin levels results from an impaired response to the insulin.

Laboratory evaluation

The procedures for performing renal function tests and the normal values they produce have been discussed.[1,2] The tests most commonly used in diagnosis and management of chronic primary renal failure are the blood urea nitrogen (BUN), creatinine, urine specific gravity, and serum inorganic phosphorus. Serum creatinine is more accurate than the BUN because it is not influenced by factors such as diet and exercise.

Moderate renal failure occurs when the kidneys cannot adequately concentrate urine (*i.e.* serial specific gravities range from 1.010 to 1.018) and creatinine levels are between 2.0 and 5.0 mg/dl. Serum creatinine levels of 5 to 10 mg/dl indicate severe renal failure that is usually refractory to treatment. Levels greater than 10 mg/dl indicate grave renal failure which is virtually always refractory to treatment. Creatinine and BUN levels can be markedly elevated in patients with obstructive uropathies or acute renal failure. But in these cases, when the cause is eliminated, the kidneys usually maintain the ability to concentrate urine, and the prognosis is much better than for cases of chronic primary renal failure with polyuria.

Laboratory evaluation of serum inorganic phosphorus is also useful in managing chronic renal failure. Animals with serum inorganic phosphorus levels between 5 and 10 mg/dl have severe renal failure. When levels become greater than 10 mg/dl, the patient's condition becomes critical and, usually, untreatable.

Treatment and management

The medical management of chronic primary renal failure includes: unlimited access to water, low-protein diets, oral administration of sodium bicarbonate, sodium chloride, multiple vitamins, anabolic steroids, calcium-vitamin D preparations and, when necessary, agents to control hyperphosphatemia. Sodium bicarbonate and sodium chloride can easily be given by sprinkling baking soda and table salt on the animal's food.

Agents to control hyperphosphatemia include aluminum hydroxide suspension (Amphojel® — Wyeth) given orally (t.i.d.) at a dose of 5 to 10 ml or aluminum hydroxide tablets (Amphojel) given at a dose of 300 mg t.i.d. with meals. These agents bind phosphate in the digestive tract, thus preventing the absorption of phosphate.

Multiple vitamins are needed to stimulate the appetite and to replace water-soluble vitamins lost because of polyuria. Anabolic steroids or an anabolic hormone such as testosterone proprionate (10 to 25 mg/day) will stimulate the bone marrow to produce erythrocytes. The action of these steroids or hormones is similar to the action of erythropoietin.

Calcium carbonate, given orally at a rate of 50 mg/lb/day, and supplemental vitamin D aid in retarding osteodystrophy. When the product of the serum calcium and serum phosphorus levels multiplied together exceeds 80, then calcification of soft tissues can occur. Low-protein diets and drugs that inhibit intestinal absorption of phosphates should be used to reduce the levels of serum phosphorus.

Low-protein diets minimize the accumulation of phosphorus, reduce the BUN, and reduce endogenous catabolism of protein. Subsequently they cause less nausea, heightened appetite, increased desire for exercise, and stabilization or improvement of the anemia. The minimum daily requirement of protein for normal dogs is 0.6 g of protein/lb of body weight. For relief of the signs of uremia in cases of chronic renal failure, dietary protein intake should be less than the minimum daily requirement. In uremic human patients, a low-protein diet contains about one-half the minimum daily requirement of protein.

Commercially available low-protein diets for

TABLE 1—Foods Used in Cases of Renal Failure*

	Protein (grams)	Energy (kcal)
Bread, toast - 1 slice	2.0	60
Butter, margarine - 1 tsp	—	40
Cake, cupcake:	2.6	130
Pound - 1 slice (2 in. x 3 in. x 5 in.)	2.1	130
Sponge - 2-in. slice	3.2	120
Cream cheese - 1 oz	2.6	106
Corn flakes - 1 cup	2.0	96
Cream, light - 1 oz	—	50
Doughnut - 1	2.1	130
Eggs, cooked - 1	7.0	120
Gravy - 1 tbsp	—	80
Ice cream - 1 oz	1.2	62
Jelly - 1 tsp	—	60
Macaroni & cheese - 1 cup	17.8	460
Milk, whole - 2 oz	2.0	40
Pancakes, wheat (4-in. dia.) - 1	1.8	60
Sweet roll (4 in. x 1 in.) - 50 g	4.2	160
Rice, cooked - 1 cup	4.2	200
Soups:		
Bouillon, consomme - 1 cup	2.0	9
Chicken - 1 cup	3.5	75
Spaghetti, cooked - 1 cup	7.4	220
Sugar, honey - 1 tsp	—	20

* Reprinted with permission from The Uremic Syndrome: Patient Evaluation and Treatment. *Comp. Cont. Ed. 1*(4); 1979.

dogs are not as restricted in protein as those used in man. Independent repeated analyses indicate Prescription Diet® k/d (Hill's Pet Products) contains 19% protein on a dry-matter basis, whereas Fit and Trim® (Purina) and Cycle 2® (Gaines) contain 18% and 20%, respectively.[3] Prescription Diet® u/d (Hill's Pet Products) appears to be the most suitable commercially available diet for patients with chronic renal failure. The product contains 8% protein on a dry-matter basis, which is still higher than is recommended for uremic dogs.[3]

Recent research indicates that low-protein diets are not beneficial during the early stages of renal disease. The decision to begin restricting protein depends on the patient's signs and the degree of renal dysfunction. Suggested guidelines for when to begin protein restriction are: when the BUN is greater than 80 mg/dl, the serum creatinine is greater than 2.5 mg/dl, or the inorganic phosphorus level is elevated.[4]

Table 1 lists foods that can be fed to patients with chronic renal failure. Owners can calculate from this list a daily diet that provides at least 35 calories/lb/day and less than 0.6 g protein/lb/day. The daily dietary intake should be divided into three feedings, each liberally sprinkled with table salt and baking soda.

REFERENCES

1. Goldston, R.T. *et al*: The Clinical Pathology Laboratory — 14: Evaluation of Renal Function — 1. *VM/SAC 76*(2):157-158; Feb. 1981.
2. Wilkes, R.D. *et al*: The Clinical Pathology Laboratory — 15: Renal Function Tests — 2. *VM/SAC 76*(3):289-291; March 1981.
3. Bovee, K.C.: Letters to the Editor. *Comp. Cont. Ed. 1*(12):884-935; Dec. 1979.
4. Bovee, K.C.: The Uremic Syndrome: Patient Evaluation and Treatment. *Comp. Cont. Ed. 1*(4):279-283; April 1979.

CHAPTER 17

Hepatic enzymology

HEPATIC FUNCTION depends on the integrity and interaction of the four anatomic subunits of the liver: 1) the hepatic parenchymal cells, 2) the biliary system, 3) the hepatic vascular system, and 4) the Kupffer or reticuloendothelial system. Hepatic disease most often involves a combination of the parenchymal cells, bile ducts, and/or vascular system, and is manifested as: 1) necrosis of the hepatic cells, 2) obstruction of the bile duct (cholestasis), and 3) hepatic atrophy or fibrosis.

The liver has tremendous functional reserve as well as the ability to regenerate its damaged cells. As much as 85% of the liver has been removed experimentally before impaired function was detected by laboratory tests.[1] There are three types of tests for evaluating hepatic disease:

1. Those that measure serum enzyme activity.
2. Those that measure bilirubin or organic dye secretion and excretion.
3. Those that measure a specific metabolism function such as plasma proteins.

Serum enzyme activity can increase as a result of necrosis or enzyme leakage from damaged hepatic cells. Overproduction of enzyme by biliary epithelial cells is the main cause of elevated serum levels of serum alkaline phosphatase (SAP).

Hepatic necrosis

Enzymes that increase in concentration in the serum after hepatic necrosis or injury to hepatic cells include: alanine aminotransferase (formerly serum glutamic pyruvic transaminase [SGPT]), aspartate aminotransferase (formerly serum glutamic oxaloacetic transaminase [SGOT]), sorbitol dehydrogenase (SDH), and arginase. The magnitude of the increase in serum levels of these enzymes relates directly to the number of affected hepatocytes and does not reflect the degree of reversibility or irreversibility of the disease process. For example, extremely high serum enzyme levels can be seen in association with shock, acute poisoning, thiacetarsamide therapy, and abdominal trauma. However, enzyme levels return to normal one to two weeks after these conditions have been eliminated. In contrast, focal necrosis from malignant neoplasia involving the liver may only cause mild elevations of serum enzyme levels.

Alanine aminotransferase (SGPT)

Alanine aminotransferase is the most liver-specific enzyme in dogs, cats, and primates and is present in large quantities in the liver of these species. (It has no diagnostic value in farm animals.) Hepatic necrosis or cell damage resulting in altered permeability of the cell causes elevations of SGPT.

Normal values for SGPT in dogs and cats range from 10 to 80 IU/liter. Serum levels of 80 to 400 IU/liter indicate moderate necrosis or enzyme leakage. Values greater than 400 IU/liter indicate severe necrosis. After hepatic necrosis and regeneration, levels of SGPT remain elevated one to three weeks.

Aspartate aminotransferase (SGOT)

Aspartate aminotransferase exists in significant quantities in the liver, skeletal muscles, and cardiac muscles of all domestic species. Necrosis of cells in any of these tissues causes elevation of SGOT. Elevated levels of SGOT in the presence of other abnormal results of liver function tests indicate that the cause of the elevated SGOT is in the liver. Elevation of SGOT in the absence of abnormal results of other liver function tests indicate the cause of the elevated SGOT is in the cardiac or skeletal muscles. Normal values for SGOT in dogs and cats range from 10 to 80 IU/liter. Hemolysis of blood samples can also cause significant elevations of SGOT.

Sorbitol dehydrogenase (SDH)

Sorbitol dehydrogenase has not been used much in small animal medicine because it gives the same information as SGPT. But, in laboratory diagnosis of diseases of farm animals, SDH is one of the most commonly used liver-specific enzymes. Elevations of SDH indicate hepatic necrosis in all species of animals.

Arginase

Arginase is a liver-specific enzyme in all domestic animals. After acute injury to the liver, serum arginase levels rise rapidly, then rapidly return to normal after the patient recovers. In contrast, SGPT levels remain elevated for up to three weeks after recovery.

Clinical and experimental data indicate that simultaneous measurement of serum arginase and SGPT in dogs with hepatic necrosis permits analysis of whether the necrosis is progressive or the liver is regenerating. High serum levels of both serum arginase and SGPT indicate continuing necrosis, whereas high levels of SGPT and normal or low levels of arginase indicate regeneration.

Cholestasis

Cholestasis can occur with or without icterus. Detection and evaluation of cholestasis is accomplished by determining SAP, serum gamma glutamyl transpeptidase (gamma-gt), and bilirubin. (The measurement of bilirubin and its conjugates in serum and urine will be discussed later.)

Serum alkaline phosphatase

Total levels of SAP are the sum of several isoenzymes of alkaline phosphatase from tissues such as liver, bone, placenta, intestinal mucosa, and renal cortex. Elevation of SAP can be caused by any space-occupying hepatic lesion and any metabolic disease or process that causes hyperlipidemia and hepatic lipidosis (*e.g.* diabetes mellitus, hypothyroidism, Cushing disease, and acute pancreatitis). Drugs that are microsomal enzyme inducers such as phenobarbital, dilantin, glucocorticoids, and adrenocorticotropic hormone can also cause increases in SAP.

Even though SAP can be found in many tissues, elevated serum levels seen clinically are entirely due to either liver or bone isoenzymes. The half-life of SAP isoenzymes of the liver and bone is about three days. The half-life of SAP isoenzymes of intestine, kidney, and placenta is only three to six minutes; therefore, in disorders of these tissues significant levels of SAP are not reached. Increases in SAP to 10 times the normal level virtually always indicate the presence of liver lesions. Recent evidence has shown that elevated SAP levels in cases of cholestasis are not a result of failure of biliary excretion but are caused by overproduction of the enzyme by the liver.

Increases of SAP involving bone isoenzymes are seen in growing dogs of the large breeds and in cases of osteomalacia, osteosarcoma, and secondary hyperparathyroidism of either renal or nutritional origin. Elevations of SAP involving hepatic isoenzymes are seen most dramatically in cases of extreme cholestasis with obstructive jaundice and in cases of steroid-induced hepatopathy.

Measurement of SAP activity has not been considered as accurate and effective a test for hepatic disease in cats as it has in dogs, because SAP activity in cats is reduced. The half-life of SAP in cats is only six hours (one-twelfth that for dogs), and the concentration of SAP in the feline liver is less than one-fourth the concentration in dogs. Normal values for total SAP in dogs is 20 to 120 IU/liter; in cats it is 10 to 80 IU/liter.

Gamma-glutamyltranspeptidase

Gamma-gt is synthetized primarily in the liver. Marked elevations of gamma-gt are seen only when the liver is diseased, making gamma-gt a liver-specific enzyme. Gamma-gt is similar to SAP, in that significantly elevated levels are seen primarily when biliary obstruction is present. Determinations for gamma-gt have not become clinically useful enough to replace SAP as the enzyme test of choice for diagnosing cholestasis.

Comments

The techniques for measuring serum levels of hepatic enzymes are available in prepared kits for use with colorimeters and spectrophotometers. Also, because these tests are so popular in human medicine, they can readily be performed by commercial laboratories that service human medicine. The tests require no conversion or standardization.

REFERENCE

1. Coles, E.H.: *Veterinary Clinical Pathology*, 2nd ed. W.B. Saunders, Philadelphia, Pa., 1974; p 192.

CHAPTER 18

Bilirubin metabolism, bromsulphalein (BSP) excretion test

THE LIVER is a complex organ that performs many metabolic functions. No single test of liver activity is sufficient for clinical assessment of most liver problems. Determinations of serum and urine bilirubin levels are among the more important laboratory tests for assessing hepatic activity. To understand these tests, a knowledge of bilirubin metabolism is essential.

Bilirubin is formed in reticuloendothelial (RE) cells, primarily through the breakdown of hemoglobin from senescent erythrocytes. Other sources of bilirubin are: intracorpuscular degradation of hemoglobin in the bone marrow and degradation of nonhemoglobin, heme-containing proteins such as myoglobin and cytochromes. Hemoglobin is absorbed into RE cells and broken down into bilirubin, iron, and globin. Iron and globin are reused by the body. Bilirubin is released into the blood where it is bound with albumin and transported to the liver.

Because it is bound with albumin, this form of bilirubin cannot be filtered by the normal renal glomerulus. The albumin-bound bilirubin is called indirect bilirubin, prehepatic bilirubin, insoluble bilirubin, or preferably, *unconjugated bilirubin*. After unconjugated bilirubin reaches the liver, it is dissociated from the carrier protein (albumin) and taken up by the hepatocytes. In the hepatocytes it is conjugated with glucuronic and sulfuric acids. This form of bilirubin is called direct bilirubin, posthepatic bilirubin, soluble bilirubin, or preferably, *conjugated bilirubin*.

Normally, after bilirubin is conjugated, most of it is released into the biliary system where it is eventually discharged into the duodenum. (A small amount does escape from the liver directly into the blood stream.) In the intestines, bacterial enzyme action converts conjugated bilirubin into urobilinogen, a colorless compound. Most of this urobilinogen is oxidized to urobilin, which imparts the characteristic brown color to feces. However, some of the urobilinogen is reabsorbed into the blood and either reexcreted by the liver or excreted into the urine as urine urobilinogen.

When the liver is in an abnormal state, *e.g.* from hepatocellular damage or biliary obstruction, the conjugated bilirubin is regurgitated back into the blood stream. This water-soluble bilirubin is filtered by the glomerulus and appears in the urine as urine bilirubin.

Serum bilirubin

Total serum bilirubin is the total measurement of both conjugated and unconjugated bilirubin in the serum. The normal range of total serum bilirubin for dogs and cats is 0.1 to 0.6 mg/dl.

The Van den Bergh test for serum bilirubin permits differentiation between conjugated and unconjugated bilirubin. In the test, a colorimeter is used to measure total bilirubin and conjugated bilirubin. The numerical difference between these values equals the unconjugated bilirubin. Because the Van den Bergh test is not sensitive enough at low concentrations to differentiate between conjugated and unconjugated bilirubin, it is not useful unless total serum bilirubin is moderately elevated.

Hyperbilirubinemia (total serum bilirubin greater than 1.0 mg/dl for dogs and cats) is recognized clinically as icterus or jaundice. Icterus or hyperbilirubinemia may be caused by excessive hemolysis, hepatocellular damage, or biliary obstruction (cholestasis). When the cause is excessive hemolysis, results of the Van den Bergh test will show greater than 60% of the total serum bilirubin to be unconjugated bilirubin. In dogs and cats, if hyperbilirubinemia is caused by cholestasis, results of the test will show greater than 60% of the total serum bilirubin to be conjugated bilirubin. Hyperbilirubinemia caused by hepatocellular disease usually results in 50% conjugated and 50% unconjugated bilirubin.

The techniques and methodology for measuring total serum bilirubin are available in prepared kits for use with colorimeters and spectrophotometers.

TABLE 1—Recommended Procedure for Detection of Bilirubin with Ictotest® *

1. Place 5 drops of urine on a square of the test mat.
2. Place a reagent tablet on the center of the moistened area of the mat.
3. Place 2 drops of water on the tablet.
4. Evaluate the test mat for a color change after 30 seconds.
5. No change or a change to pink or red indicates lack of bilirubin. A positive result is indicated by blue or purple. The speed and intensity of color development is proportional to the degree of bilirubinuria.
6. Color changes affecting the tablet or changes occurring after a lapse of 30 seconds should not be interpreted as positive or negative results.

*Ames Co., Div. Miles Laboratories, Inc., Elkhart, Ind. 46515.

TABLE 2—Recommended Procedure for Detection of Bilirubinuria with Reagent Stick Tests*

1. Immerse the reagent pad of the strip in the urine sample and remove it immediately. Tap the edge of the strip against the side of the container to remove excess urine.
2. After 20 seconds, compare the color of the reagent pad to the color scale provided by the manufacturer.
3. Pale lemon indicates a negative reaction. Positive reactions are indicated by light tan (+ or 0.3 mg/dl), dark tan (+ + or 0.5 mg/dl), and light brown (+ + + or 1.0 mg/dl). Careful comparisons are recommended because color changes may be subtle.
4. Urine that is concentrated or discolored may be unsuitable for evaluation by this method. Questionable results can be verified with a different test method.

*Ictostix®, Multistix® (Ames Co., Div. Miles Laboratories, Inc., Elkhart, Ind. 46516.

TABLE 3—Recommended Procedure for Detection of Bilirubinuria with Chemstrips*

1. Immerse the reagent pad of the strip in a fresh urine sample and remove it immediately.
2. Tap the edge of the strip against the side of the container to remove excess urine.
3. After 30 to 60 seconds, compare the color of the reagent pad to the color scale provided by the manufacturer.
4. No change indicates a negative reaction. A change of the test zone from white to beige-pink indicates bilirubinuria. Varying shades of beige-pink to pale red-violet indicate slight (+ or 0.5 mg/dl), moderate (+ + or 1.0 mg/dl), and heavy (+ + + or 2.0 mg/dl) bilirubinuria.

*Bio-Dynamics, Indianapolis, Ind. 46206.

TABLE 4—Procedure for Bromsulphalein (BSP)* Excretion Test

1. The animal should be fasted and should not be receiving medication.
2. BSP is injected intravenously at a rate of 5 mg/kg. (BSP is a tissue irritant if injected perivascularly.)
3. After exactly 30 minutes, a 10-ml blood sample is obtained from another vein and placed into a plain or heparinized vacutainer.
4. The blood sample is centrifuged to obtain 2 ml of serum/plasma. It is then submitted to a commercial laboratory for colorimetric analysis.

*Bromsuphalein (BSP), Hynson, Wescott and Dunning, Inc., Baltimore, Maryland: 1-800 638-1532.

Also, the test can be performed by commercial laboratories specializing in human medicine. The tests require no special conversion.

Urine bilirubin

Conjugated bilirubin escapes in small amounts from the normal liver, and in large amounts if hepatocellular disease or cholestasis is present. This bilirubin will appear in the urine. The renal threshold for clearance of conjugated bilirubin varies from species to species. It is low in dogs and relatively high in cats. Normal dogs with concentrated urine (specific gravity greater than 1.040) can show trace amounts of bilirubinuria.

Results of recent studies have shown that the canine kidney can form small amounts of bilirubin from filtered hemoglobin and can also conjugate bilirubin with glucuronic acid acid in the renal tubule cells.[1] This capacity is greater in males than in females. In a retrospective survey of 1000 canine urine samples, 77.3% of bilirubin-positive samples were from males and 22.7% from females.[1] Abnormally large quantities of bilirubin in the urine may be conjugated bilirubin from hemolysis or may result from increased serum levels of conjugated bilirubin caused by hepatocellular disease or cholestasis.

Tests for bilirubin in the urine can be performed with reagent sticks such as Ictostix® or Multistix® (Ames), with reagent tablets such as Ictotest® (Ames), or with Chemstrips® 6, 7, and 8 (Biodynamics). Procedures for performing these tests are outlined in Tables 1-3.

Urine urobilinogen

Urine urobilinogen can be detected by a semiquantitative, dipstick test to help identify patients with obstructive jaundice. The presence of urobilinogen in the urine is dependent on the secretion and release of bile into the intestines. The absence of urobilinogen in the urine is suggestive of a total biliary obstruction, rarely seen in clinical cases. Excessive amounts of urobilinogen may indicate hemolytic disease.

Known causes of increased urine urobilinogen are hemolysis, constipation, and chronic hepatic disease. Urobilinogen is unstable in acid urine and in light, so tests for urine urobilinogen should be done soon after the urine is collected.

Bromsulphalein (BSP)® excretion test

When injected into the blood stream, BSP, an organic dye, is removed by the liver at a rate that reflects the liver's ability to metabolize similar organic dyes. When hepatic function or circulation is impaired by disease, the dye is retained in the circulation for an abnormal time. Normal BSP retention for dogs is less then 5% and in cats less than 10% at 30 minutes postinjection.

Because BSP rapidly binds with albumin when injected, the BSP excretion rate is also dependent on the concentration of plasma protein. Hypoproteinemic animals bind less of the BSP and subsequently, the liver removes the BSP faster. Reduced hepatic function causes prolonged retention of BSP, but when associated with a hypoproteinemia that increases BSP excretion, the end result may be a BSP clearance in the normal range. Measurement of BSP retention time does not yield any additional useful information in animals that are already icteric. This is because the abnormal retention of bilirubin already reflects an impaired capacity of the liver to take up, conjugate, and secrete an organic dye.

The BSP retention time is determined by measuring the plasma concentration of BSP 30 minutes after the dye is injected intravenously. The amount of BSP given is 5 mg/kg. Animals should be fasted and should not be receiving medication at the time of the test. The procedure for the BSP retention test is outlined in Table 4.

REFERENCE

1. Osborne, C.A. *et al*: Clinical Significance of Bilirubinuria. *Compend. Cont. Ed.* 2(11):897-902; Nov. 1980.

CHAPTER 19

Protein metabolism and blood ammonia tests

THE LIVER is the primary source of plasma protein. All albumin; 80% of serum globulins; prothrombin; fibrinogen; most clotting factors; lipoproteins; glycoproteins; and mucoproteins are produced in the liver. Plasma protein levels indicate the relative balance between protein synthesis and catabolism. Nonhepatic factors may be involved in controlling this balance.

When used in conjunction with other tests for evaulating liver function, levels of total plasma protein and protein fractions can aid in confirming a specific disease. Changes in the different fractions of plasma protein are better indicators of liver disease than total plasma protein levels. For example, an increase in globulin can mask a decrease in albumin unless the fractions are measured.

Total protein (albumin and globulins)

Total protein levels become elevated when relative polycythemia occurs. Total protein increases proportionately to the amount of hemoconcentration. A rise in the gamma globulin level occurs in response to antigenic stimulation caused by infectious and suppurative diseases.

Reduced total protein levels result from inhibited production of protein, malnutrition, malabsorption, liver disease, and neoplasia. Acute and chronic loss of blood lowers total protein levels. In cases of acute blood loss, extravascular fluid dilutes plasma proteins. Upon recovery from one or more of these conditions, the total protein level gradually returns to normal.

Chronic loss of protein into the gastrointestinal system by exudation (protein-losing enteropathy) reduces total plasma protein levels. Albumin and small amounts of globulins are lost through the kidneys because of glomerular damage, resulting in lowered albumin levels and a low level of total plasma protein. Parasitism reduces levels of total protein and albumin, but increases the concentration of gamma globulin.

A low albumin level and an elevated globulin level are often seen in patients with liver damage. Diffuse and chronic liver disease reduces albumin concentrations. Albumin levels decline gradually because the half-life of albumin is 12 to 18 days. In extremely chronic cases of liver disease, albumin levels approach 1 to 2 g/dl. The normal range of plasma albumin for dogs and cats is 3.1 to 4 g/dl.[1]

Acute hepatitis does not significantly alter albumin levels. Serum albumin levels are lowered in cases of subacute hepatitis, hepatic fibrosis, and hepatic neoplasia. As with total protein levels, albumin levels are reduced by malnutrition, malabsorption, infections, renal disease, and protein-losing enteropathies. Edema, ascites, and hydrothorax commonly occur when albumin levels are depressed to between 1 and 2 g/dl.[2]

Globulins carry various lipids, lipid-soluble hormones and vitamins (alpha and beta globulins), and gamma globulins (primarily associated with antibodies). Although nonspecific, gamma globulins are elevated in cases of diffuse hepatic fibrosis and hepatitis. Certain tumors, acute and chronic bacterial infections, and diseases of the reticuloendothelial system cause elevations in the levels of gamma globulins. Alpha-2 globulin is nonspecific and unimportant in hepatic evaluation. Peaks in the level of beta-1 globulin are associated with neoplastic conditions. In all other hepatic conditions, the level of beta-1 globulin is reduced. Beta-2 globulin levels are elevated in patients with jaundice and hepatic cirrhosis.

Usually, more information is gained from albumin and total globulin levels than from total protein levels only. When globulin levels are abnormal, examination of protein fractions may reveal the reason for the alteration.

Total plasma protein can be measured by refractometric, Biuret, and Kjeldahl methods. The simple, precise refractometric method is outlined in Table 1. The simplest chemical quantitative analytic method is the Biuret method. In this method, which measures peptide links that characterize protein, copper sulfate reagent tablets are used. The method can also be used to quantitate albumin and globulin. The Kjeldahl method measures total serum or plasma nitrogen, which reflects the level of protein. However, this method is complicated and is performed in few hospitals.

Albumin is commonly measured by means of a dye-binding technique used in many automated chemistry instruments (SMA-12-Technicon) and blood analyzer systems (BMI/Ames).

Paper- or cellulose-acetate electrophoresis divides protein into five measured components. With immunoelectrophoresis, 30 or more fractions can be separated. Both techniques are done in many human hospitals and commercial laboratories.

TABLE 1—Method for Measuring Total Protein with a Refractometer

1. Place a drop of serum or plasma on the glass prism of the refractometer.
2. Place cover over drop of serum or plasma and apply gentle pressure to spread drop into a thin layer.
3. With certain newer models light is not required for reading the scale. If light is required, hold the instrument toward bright light.
4. Take a reading at junction of lighter and darker fields.
5. Adjust eyepiece to bring the junction or reading into sharp contrast.
6. Use a conversion table if the refractometer does not have a scale in g/dl. With most models total protein is read in grams and urine specific gravity is read directly. A refractive index or total-solids scale is converted by using a table.
7. The temperature of the sample or refractometer will alter the test readings. Certain models compensate for this.
8. Cloudy, lipemic serum or serum with free hemoglobin will give high values.

Prothrombin

Prothrombin is produced by the liver, and measurement of prothrombin time can be used in evaluating certain liver conditions. Severe hepatocellular disease and prolonged obstruction of the bile duct that results in hypovitaminosis K will prolong prothrombin time. A simple way to differentiate these abnormalities is to measure prothrombin time 24 to 48 hours after an aqueous injection of vitamin K is given. If the bile duct is obstructed, the prothrombin time will be normal. Normal prothrombin time ranges from 7.4 to 8.6 seconds.[3] The importance of prolonged prothrombin time in evaluating liver disease is controversial.

Prolonged prothrombin time occurs as a result of dietary deficiency of vitamin K, malabsorption of vitamin K, and diseases such as infectious canine hepatitis and diffuse hepatic fibrosis. Dicumarol, an anticoagulant, will also prolong prothrombin time. Prothrombin time can be determined by the one-stage prothrombin time test shown in Table 2.

Blood ammonia

Blood ammonia concentrations provide an indication of hepatic function. Most of the ammonia in blood is produced in the intestines from degradation of protein and by bacteria splitting urea into ammonia. A normal liver efficiently removes this ammonia from the blood. Analysis for blood ammonia should be done several hours after feeding or after ammonium chloride (ammonia tolerance test) is given orally. This increases the chance of detecting hyperammonemia.

Samples for blood ammonia determinations should be taken without exposing the sample to air. A heparinized vacutainer is filled as full as possible and air is removed to create a slight vacuum in the tube. The sample is immediately placed in an ice bath. Plasma must be removed from the blood

Table 2—Test for One-Stage Prothrombin Time[3]

Reagents:

1. Thromboplastin (This reagent is commercially prepared, usually in the form of a suspension of acetone-dried extract of brain tissue.)
2. Calcium chloride 0.02 molar (Many preparations are available in which the thromboplastin and calcium are mixed and ready for use.)

Procedure:

1. Place test tubes in a warm water bath.
2. Add 0.2 ml of thromboplastin-calcium mixture to each tube, or add 0.1 ml thromboplastin and 0.1 ml calcium chloride.
3. Allow tubes to warm for about 30 seconds.
4. Taking one tube at a time, add 0.1 ml of sample plasma by blowing it quickly into the thromboplastin mixture. Start stop watch at the same time.
5. While continuously and gently agitating the tube, leave it in the water bath for 10 seconds.
6. Remove tube, hold it in front of a bright light, and tilt it slightly every second until a clot appears. Stop the watch after a clot appears.
7. Test each sample twice and average results.
8. Include a normal plasma control with each batch. Results are reported in seconds. The control time should also be recorded.

within 30 minutes. If necessary the plasma can be refrigerated for as long as three hours. Plasma refrigerated for up to seven hours will show a substantial increase in blood ammonia.[4]

Blood ammonia is determined by several methods, but the method of choice involves the use of a binding resin. Reagents to conduct this test are available commercially (Hyland Blood Ammonia Test-Travenol Laboratories). Care must be taken to prevent ammonia contamination of samples. Glassware should be washed with ammonia-free water and detergents.

Commercial laboratories usually perform the test more accurately than the practitioner. A control sample should be run concurrently with the test sample. When the resin-binding technique is used, normal peripheral levels of blood ammonia for dogs and cats are less than 50 μg/L. Another method used extensively by commercial laboratories is based on an enzymatic conversion of alpha-ketogluterate to glutomate in the presence of ammonia. Normal blood ammonia levels for dogs and cats tested this way range from 60 to 120 μg/dl.

Ammonia tolerance test

The ammonia tolerance test increases the chance of detecting hyperammonemia in animals in which hepatic disease is questionable. A blood sample is taken, as described, for a prechallenge blood ammonia level. Ammonium chloride at a rate of 100 mg/kg (maximum of 3 g) is dissolved in water and given orally via a stomach tube. A postchallenge blood sample for determination of blood ammonia is taken 30 minutes later. Because normal animals can remove the ammonia given, little increase should be seen in the postchallenge blood sample.

Hepatic encephalopathy

Clinical signs of hepatic encephalopathy appear when metabolism of amino acids and ammonia are abnormal.[5,6] Clinical signs range from hepatic coma, seizures, and bizarre behavioral changes, to nonspecific signs related to the central nervous system such as listlessness, depression, vomiting, diarrhea, and polydipsia. Pathophysiology of the condition involves changes in amino acid composition of the plasma and the inability of the liver to remove ammonia and mercaptans from the plasma.

Ammonia is formed from protein metabolism and urea-splitting bacteria. Mercaptan is formed from deamination of sulfur-containing amino acids, especially methionine. Methionine (present in most lipotrophics) given orally can cause signs of hepatic encephalopathy to worsen, producing coma in dogs.[7] The changes in concentration of amino acids are caused by inability of the liver to metabolize aromatic amino acids (phenylalanine, tyrosine, and tryptophan), which causes their levels to be elevated in the plasma. This is further complicated by a decrease in plasma levels of branched-chained amino acids caused by an increase in plasma levels of their regulatory hormones (insulin, glucogon, and catecholamine) in cases of liver failure.

Management of hepatic encephalopathy involves control of urea-splitting bacteria with nonabsorbable antibiotics, replacement of urea-splitting bacteria with nonurease-producing *Lactobacillus*, feeding patients a diet high in carbohydrates and low in protein, and acidifying and increasing transit time of the colon contents. Lactulose (Cephalac—Merrill Laboratories) is a disaccharide not absorbed by the small intestines. The drug ferments in the colon, causing acidification of the colon contents and osmotic influx of water into the colon. Thus, colonic transit time is increased. Acidification of colonic contents reduces the conversion of nonionized (absorbable) ammonia (NH_3 −) to the ionized (relatively unabsorbable) ammonium ion (NH_4 +).

REFERENCES

1. Ettinger, S.J.: *Textbook of Veterinary Internal Medicine*, vol. 2. W.B. Saunders, Philadephia, Pa., 1975.
2. Benjamin, M.M.: *Outline of Veterinary Clinical Pathology*, 3rd ed. The Iowa State University Press, Ames, Iowa, 1978.
3. Coles, E.H.: *Veterinary Clinical Pathology*, 2nd ed. W.B. Saunders, Philadelphia, Pa., 1974.
4. Mondzac, A. *et al*: An Enzymatic Determination of Ammonia in Biological Fluids. *J. Lab. Clin. Med.* *66*:526; 1965.
5. Ewing, G.O. *et al*: Hepatic Insufficiency Associated with Congenital Anomalies of the Portal Vein in Dog. JAAHA 10:453-476; 1974.
6. Strombeck, D.R. *et al*: Hyperammonemia and Hepatic Encephalopathy in the Dog. *JAVMA* *166*:1105-1108; 1975.
7. Merion, G.E. *et al*: Methionine-induced Hepatic Coma in Dogs. *Am. J. Surg.* *130*:41-46; 1975.

from intestinal malabsorption.

6. If hyperinsulinism (beta-cell tumor) is present, blood glucose levels peak at lower than normal values and return to hypoglycemic levels after one to two hours.

Intravenous glucose tolerance test

1. Administer 0.5 g glucose/lb.
2. In normal animals, blood glucose should return to base line values within 90 minutes.
3. In cases of diabetes mellitus, blood glucose levels fail to return to base line values within 90 minutes.
4. Cats should be given 0.5 g glucose/kg. In normal cats, blood glucose levels return to base line values 120 to 180 minutes after administration. Diabetes mellitus is diagnosed if glucose levels don't return to base line values within 180 minutes.

Glucagon response test

Administration of glucagon causes the release of insulin. An exaggerated response occurs when a functional beta-cell tumor is present.

1. A blood glucose test is performed after a 12-hour fast.
2. Give 0.03 mg glucagon/kg intravenously.
3. Blood glucose levels will be lower than normal in affected animals.
4. If a functional beta-cell tumor is present, hypoglycemia (<50 mg/dl) occurs 45 to 90 minutes after glucagon is given. Normal animals show a slower decline in blood glucose values.
5. Normal or unresponsive dogs with beta-cell tumors do not become hypoglycemic.

REFERENCES

1. Ettinger, S.J.: *Textbook of Veterinary Internal Medicine*, vol. 2. W.B. Saunders, Philadelphia, Pa., 1975.
2. Duncan, J.R.; Prasse, K.E.: *Veterinary Laboratory Medicine, Clinical Pathology*. Iowa State University Press, Ames, Iowa, 1977.

CHAPTER 22

Diabetes mellitus

Diabetes mellitus is associated with abnormal lipid, protein, and carbohydrate metabolism. Insulin deficiency at the cellular level initiates the disease process, resulting in hyperglycemia and glucosuria (the most common clinical pathologic abnormalities occurring as a result of diabetes mellitus). Growth hormone, epinephrine, cortisol, and glucagon may cause blood glucose levels to elevate and aid in the development of diabetes mellitus.

An animal presented with polydipsia, polyphagia, and polyuria should be evaluated for diabetes mellitus. Normal blood glucose values in dogs range from 60 to 100 mg/dl;[1] values for cats are slightly higher. In the absence of complicating factors, a blood glucose value greater than 150 mg/dl is diagnostic of diabetes mellitus.[1] Postprandial absorption of glucose, stress, glucocorticoids, adrenocorticotropic hormone, estrogens, and progesterones may cause hyperglycemia. In patients with Cushing disease, a mild rise in blood glucose is noted. In stressed cats, blood glucose levels may rise significantly to 350 mg/dl.

A complete blood count (CBC), urinalysis, and biochemistry profile should be done for animals suspected of having diabetes. The results will help confirm the diagnosis and aid in determining the extent of treatment.

Colorimetric techniques are routinely used to test blood glucose levels, and Diastix® and Clinitest® (Ames) sticks are used to detect glucosuria. In some breeds (*e.g.* Norwegian Elkhound and Basenji), glucosuria can be a result of primary renal disease. To rule out this possibility, hyperglycemia and glucosuria should be present simultaneously.

For suspect diabetic animals with blood glucose levels between 120 and 170 mg/dl, an oral glucose tolerance test is indicated.[2] Normal animals will reach a peak blood glucose level within one hour and return to the baseline level within three hours. Overt diabetes mellitus may result from any stress.

In patients with diabetes mellitus, fat metabolism increases, causing lipemia and elevated serum glutamic-pyruvic transaminase and alkaline phosphatase levels due to fat infiltration of the liver. As fat infiltration continues, the liver becomes palpable and enlarged. This is the most common radiographic abnormality seen in patients with diabetes mellitus. Continued hyperglycemia can cause glomerular damage and result in proteinuria. Urinalysis is done to evaluate the extent of damage.

Treatment

Isophane (NPH) insulin (U100) is the routine form of insulin used for maintenance or control of hyperglycemia in dogs and cats (*Table 1*). Insulin should be refrigerated. Before the injection, a vial of NPH insulin should be rolled gently between the palms of the hands for thorough mixing.

When given subcutaneously, NPH insulin begins to act in three hours and peaks in 6 to 10 hours. Feedings should correspond to these times. One-fourth of the daily caloric requirement should be fed after insulin is given, and the remaining three-

TABLE 1—Types of Insulin

	Hours after Administration		
Types	Effects begin	Peak blood level	Duration of effects
Regular	¼	2-4	6-8
NPH	3	6-10	18-24
Lente	3	8-12	12-24
PZI	3-4	14-20	24-36

TABLE 2—Insulin Dosage Change for 20-lb Dog

Percent of Urine Glucose on Dipstix	Insulin Change
2%	Increase 1 unit
1%	Increase ½ unit
0.5%	Increase ½ unit
0.1-0.25%	Repeat previous day's dosage
Negative	Decrease 1 unit

fourths 10 hours after the injection. Anorectic animals are given insulin only after they eat in the morning.

NPH insulin should be given at a dosage of 0.5 to 1.0 units/kg, subcutaneously every 24 hours (modified as needed). Cats are more sensitive to insulin and require a smaller dosage (0.25 to 0.5 units/kg every 24 hours, subcutaneously, modified as needed).[1]

Although most owners who understand the procedure to control diabetes mellitus take their responsibility seriously, the veterinarian should stress careful control of blood glucose. Overdosage of insulin can lead to a hypoglycemic crisis, and underdosage will eventually lead to cataracts, polydipsia, polyuria and possibly, ketoacidosis. To prevent over- or underdosing, owners should routinely measure urine glucose and periodically adjust insulin dosage as necessary (*Table 2*).[1]

Initially, diabetic animals should be hospitalized until the insulin dosage is determined. Exercise and caloric intake should be constant. Usually, animals exercise and eat more at home, so the dosage must be readjusted. It is best to start with a low insulin dosage to prevent hypoglycemia. While an animal is hospitalized, blood glucose levels should be evaluated before administration of insulin and the evening meal. The dosage of NPH insulin is then adjusted according to the blood glucose levels found on follow-up examinations of blood samples taken in the afternoon.

Clients should check urine glucose values in the morning. To maintain control, the blood glucose level is kept around the renal threshold of approximately 175 mg/dl. At this level, a trace to one-plus (+) level of glucosuria is noted. This gives the owner knowledge of the blood glucose level and helps prevent overdose of insulin.

If excessive glucosuria is persistent even with increased insulin dosages, the administration, mixing, or storage of insulin should be checked. Care should be taken if insulin dosage exceeds 1 U/lb body weight. Hypoglycemia can precipitate counterregulatory mechanisms that increase blood glucose levels. If this occurs, the insulin dosage should be reduced. Lente or protamine-zinc insulin may have to be used in some patients when the duration of NPH insulin is insufficient. In some animals NPH insulin has to be given twice daily.

If hypoglycemia occurs, owners should rub honey or syrup on their pets' buccal membranes. A blood glucose test should be done on any diabetic animal showing central nervous system disturbances.

Small dogs should receive 75 kcal/kg and large dogs 55 kcal/kg daily. The number of kcal should be reduced as an animal loses weight. Intact females should be ovariohysterectomized because estrus, pregnancy, and pseudopregnancy can cause resistance to insulin.

Ketoacidosis

Ketoacidosis is a common and severe complication of diabetes mellitus. Animals presented with anorexia, vomiting, diarrhea, lethargy, and possibly Kussmaul breathing, are suspect ketoacidotic. Clinical signs include depression, coma, weakness, acetone breath, fever, icterus, or shock. Clinical pathologic data helpful in monitoring the severe ketoacidotic patient include CBC, urinalysis, total protein, blood glucose, blood urea nitrogen, amylase, lipase, sodium, potassium, chloride, and blood gases (pH, PCO_2, PO_2, and HCO_3).[1]

Pancreatitis is the most common complication of ketoacidosis and the most common cause of death. For this reason, serum amylase and lipase levels should be obtained; levels greater than two times normal are suggestive of pancreatitis.

Treatment of the diabetic ketoacidotic patient includes fluids (lactated Ringer solution or 0.9% sodium chloride), electrolytes (mainly sodium and potassium), regular insulin (intravenous continuous infusion method), and possibly alkalizing agents. Continuous monitoring of laboratory values during therapy is indicated. Most values should be obtained every two to six hours until the patient's condition stabilizes. An intramuscular technique of administering a small dose of regular insulin hourly until blood glucose levels return to less than 250 mg/dl has been described.[3]

Islet cell tumors

Another endocrine abnormality that causes low blood glucose levels is the islet cell tumor. Functional islet cell tumors are rare in dogs, but are seen in Boxer, Poodle, and Terrier breeds. Clinical signs are similar to those seen in cases of hypoglycemia (weakness, ataxia, collapse, muscle tremors, and convulsions).

A tentative diagnosis is based on the Whipple triad (neurologic signs with hypoglycemia, fasting blood glucose levels below 40 mg/dl, and improvement by feeding glucose).[1] Other laboratory data are required to help differentiate islet cell tumors from other causes of hypoglycemia such as hypopituitarism, Addison disease, hypothyroidism, and disorders of the liver. Although it is considered the treatment of choice, surgery is only palliative.

REFERENCES

1. Feldman, E.C.: Diabetes Mellitus, In *Current Veterinary Therapy* (R.W. Kirk, Ed.). W.B. Saunders, Philadelphia, Pa., 1980.
2. Wilkes, R.D. *et al*: The Clinical Pathology Laboratory-21: The Pancreas-1: Evaluating Blood Glucose. *VM/SAC* 76(9):1275-1278; 1981.
3. Chastain, C.B.: Nichols, C.E.: Low-Dose Intramuscular Insulin Therapy for Diabetic Ketoacidosis in Dogs. *JAVMA* 178(6):561-564; 1981.

CHAPTER 23

Exocrine pancreatic diseases, acute pancreatitis

Exocrine pancreatic disease can range from incurable neoplasia to acute, hemorrhagic, necrotizing pancreatitis to a relatively benign, chronic insufficiency. A basic understanding of the anatomic and pathophysiology mechanisms of exocrine pancreatic diseases facilitates diagnosis and treatment.

The pancreas is a v-shaped gland with two coarse lobes. It lies in the right and left cranial quadrants of the abdomen.[1] The exocrine secretions pass into the duodenum by various duct systems, depending on the species.

In dogs, the main pancreatic duct (ventral duct) enters at the minor duodenal papilla, and the minor pancreatic duct (dorsal duct) enters the duodenum near the bile duct. Each pancreatic duct has a sphincter. Normal canine pancreatic juice has a pH of 8.0 to 8.3 and a specific gravity of 1.010 to 1.018. It contains proteolytic, amylolytic, and lipolytic enzymes. Levels of bicarbonate in normal canine pancreatic juice are higher than plasma levels. Levels of sodium, potassium, and chloride are about the same as plasma levels. In normal dogs, 25 ml/lb/day of pancreatic juice is produced.

The feline pancreatic duct and bile duct enter the duodenum via a common orifice at the major duodenal papilla. This explains why icterus occurs in cats with acute, hemorrhagic, necrotic pancreatitis. Few cats have a second pancreatic duct.

The pancreatic enzymes are synthesized by the acinar cells of the pancreas. The major proteolytic enzymes are trypsinogen, chymotrypsinogen, and procarboxypeptidase A and B. These enzymes are produced in the proenzyme (inactive) form.

Trypsinogen is activated to trypsin by enterokinase, which is produced by the duodenal mucosa. Trypsin then activates other proteolytic enzymes, which split proteins into peptones, peptides, and polypeptides. Lipase, the lipolytic enzyme, is secreted in its active form. In the presence of bile and an alkaline pH, lipase breaks triglycerides into glycerol and fatty acids. Amylase is also secreted in its active form; it hydrolyzes polysaccharides into monosaccharides and disaccharides.

Pathophysiology of pancreatitis

The basic pathologic process of pancreatitis is autodigestion resulting from destruction of cell membranes with subsequent release of proteolytic and lipolytic enzymes. There are two forms of active pancreatitis: interstitial edematous and hemorrhagic necrotizing.

There are many theories about the causes of pancreatic inflammation. Prerequisites for the condition are: obstructed pancreatic ducts and an actively secreting gland. These factors cause increased intraductal pressure, resulting in elevated pressure within the pancreas, passage of enzymes into the interstitial pancreatic tissue, and autodigestion.

The autodigestion process is primarily related to the activation by trypsin of other enzymes such as elastase and phospholipase. Elastase destroys the elastic fibers in the pancreatic arterioles, resulting in hemorrhage and tissue ischemia. Phospholipase destroys pancreatic cellular membranes, causing the release of more enzymes and continuation of the autodigestion cycle.

The pancreas releases a peptide myocardial depressant that has a negative inotropic effect on the heart. This leads to further hypovolemic shock.

Diagnosis of acute pancreatitis

Acute pancreatitis occurs with greatest frequency in middle-aged obese dogs, usually after ingestion of a large, fatty meal. In patients with this condition, deep palpation of the upper right quadrant usually reveals evidence of pain. Vomiting and bloating associated with aerophagia secondary to nausea are also frequently observed.

Laboratory findings

Serum amylase

Among the many methods of determining serum amylase activity, most are either saccharogenic or amyloclastic (iodometric). When serum amylase is measured by saccharogenic methods, maltase (present in normal canine serum) artificially elevates serum amylase levels. Therefore, in dogs, amyloclastic methods are preferred.

Most colorimeters have test kits available for determining serum amylase by the amyloclastic method. The normal serum amylase level for dogs can range as high as 1,000 IU/liter. Values of serum amylase activity up to twice normal are often associated with nonpancreatic diseases such as enteritis and renal failure.

Plasma amylase activity greater than 3,000 to 6,000 IU/liter is usually considered diagnostic for acute pancreatitis. Levels of 2,000 to 3,000 IU/liter suggest pancreatic disease, whereas values less than 2,000 IU/liter probably result from nonpancreatic problems. Determination of plasma amylase activity has not been shown to be useful for diagnosing pancreatitis in cats.[2]

Serum lipase

Measurement of serum lipase is the most important way to evaluate dogs with pancreatic disease. Pancreatitis causes a substantial increase in plasma levels of serum lipase, which is not known to be elevated significantly by any other disease.

Normal canine serum lipase activity ranges from 0 to 250 IU/liter. Values for dogs with pancreatitis are usually increased three- to fourfold. Determining serum lipase activity is more difficult than determining amylase activity.

In cats, measurement of plasma lipase levels is not always diagnostic.[3] Hyperlipasemia is diagnostic for pancreatitis in cats, but normal lipase activity does not rule out the disease.

In many laboratories, test procedures for serum amylase and serum lipase activity are not expressed in IU/liter. Normal values for these tests depend on the individual laboratory methods. For these reasons, normal values should be established within each laboratory.

Other abnormalities commonly found in patients with acute pancreatitis are hypercholesterolemia, neutrophilic leukocytosis, and hypocalcemia.

Treatment and management of acute pancreatitis

The best treatment for acute pancreatitis is placing the pancreas at physiologic rest by reducing the secretion of enzymes. This is done by ensuring that the patient receives no food or water orally. Normal fluid balance can be maintained with intravenous fluids. When clinical signs improve, carbohydrates can be reintroduced. Later, bland foods and high-quality proteins can gradually be added to the diet. Dietary control is important after the animal is dismissed from the hospital. Low-fat commercial or prescription diets are preferred.

The value of using drugs, such as anticholinergics, to inhibit pancreatic secretion is questionable. Because secretion ceases in the acutely inflamed pancreas that is not stimulated gastrically, anticholinergics may be unnecessary. They have not been shown to be useful in treating pancreatitis and may contribute to the development of complications.[4] Inflammation often extends from the pancreas to the stomach and small intestine, causing a loss of normal motility. Anticholinergics further reduce motility, thus precipitating ileus.

Cimetidine (Tagamet® —SmithKline & French) given at a dosage of 100 mg to 300 mg three times daily inhibits production of gastric acid. The drug is a histamine-2 antagonist, thus providing some of the benefits of anticholinergics but none of the disadvantages. Pancreatic circulation and hypovolemic shock can be treated with intravenous lactated Ringer solution. To bring the pH to 7.0 and provide a readily available alkali source, 12 mEq of sodium bicarbonate can be added to each liter of lactated Ringer's solution. Heparin given subcutaneously at a rate of 50 units/lb twice daily helps prevent disseminated intravascular coagulation, which occurs in patients with acute hemorrhagic necrotizing pancreatitis.

Relief of pain is important for the general well being of the animal. The analgesic of choice is Demerol® (Winthrop) at a dose of 2.5 to 5 mg/lb intramuscularly or subcutaneously. Morphine should be avoided because it causes spasms of the sphincter of the pancreatic duct and increases intraductal pressure. The use of corticosteroids is generally contraindicated, except in cases of severe shock. Corticosteriods cause hyperplasia of the pancreatic ductular epithelium and increase the viscosity of pancreatic secretion. They have been shown to induce pancreatitis in some animals.

The appropriate use of antibiotics in cases of acute pancreatitis is important.[5] Treatment must be directed against both anaerobes and aerobes. Procaine penicillin G given at a rate of 20,000 units/lb intramuscularly once daily is effective against most anaerobes. Kanamycin given intramuscularly at a dose of 2.5 mg/lb twice daily is effective against most aerobes.[6]

Vomiting in patients with acute pancreatitis is best controlled with intramuscular Thorazine® (SmithKline & French) at a dosage of 0.5 mg/lb twice daily. Like other tranquilizers, it has hypotensive properties and should be used cautiously in hypovolemic patients. Thorazine appears to be the least hypotensive of the tranquilizers that have antiemetic activity.

REFERENCES

1. Miller, M.: *Anatomy of the Dog.* W.B. Saunders, Philadelphia, Pa., 1964.
2. Strombeck, D.R.: *Small Animal Gastroenterology.* Stonegate Publishing, Davis, Calif., 1979.
3. Duffell, S.J.: Some Aspects of Pancreatic Disease in the Cat. *J. Sm. Anim. Prac.* *16*:365-374; 1975.
4. Soergel, K.H.: Medical Treatment of Acute Pancreatitis. What is the Evidence? *Gastroent.* *74*:620-628; 1978.
5. Schiller, W.R. *et al*: A Review of Experimental Pancreatitis. *J. Surg. Res.* *16*:69-90; 1974.
6. Howes, R. *et al*: Evaluation of Prophylactic Antibiotics in Acute Pancreatitis. *J. Surg. Res.* *18*:197-200; 1975.

CHAPTER 24

Exocrine pancreatic insufficiency

EXOCRINE PANCREATIC insufficiency results from repeated attacks of acute pancreatitis with progressive destruction of glandular tissue. No specific causes have been identified, but the chronic disease is thought to be a scarring and/or smoldering phase of the acute necrotic process in animals surviving the initial attack.[1] Exocrine pancreatic insufficiency is commonly seen in dogs but only rarely in cats.

History and physical examination

Patients with the condition typically are emaciated and have a voracious appetite. Their stools are voluminous, clay-colored, greasy, and loose. Owners frequently report coprophagia.

The feces may contain large quantities of undigested fat, starch, and protein. Undigested fat irritates the colon, often causing diarrhea. A deficiency of pancreatic lipase is the primary factor responsible for this malabsorption of fats.[2] Deficiencies in pancreatic amylase and proteolytic enzymes do not contribute significantly to the emaciation.

In patients with exocrine pancreatic insufficiency, more than 85% of the capability to produce pancreatic enzymes is lost.[3] Test results indicate that dogs can lose 80% of their normal pancreatic acinar tissue and still retain normal digestive function.[4]

A diagnosis of exocrine pancreatic insufficiency is based not only on history and clinical signs, but also on the exclusion of other factors leading to emaciation such as dietary insufficiency; endoparasitism; intestinal malabsorption; and chronic renal, cardiac, and hepatic disease.

Examination of feces

To rule out occult endoparasitism, numerous fecal flotations should be performed for dogs suspected of having exocrine pancreatic insufficiency. Direct smears of feces should be stained and examined for excess neutral and/or split fats (steatorrhea), starch (amylorrhea), and undigested muscle fibers (creatorrhea). The procedure for detecting steatorrhea is outlined in Table 1 and the procedure for detecting amylorrhea and creatorrhea is shown in Table 2.

A fecal enzyme test (gelatin tube or radiographic film) to detect trypsin activity should be done (*Tables 3 & 4*). This test should be repeated on three different samples. To ensure accurate results, both positive and negative controls should be done.

Absorption tests

Absorption tests are indicated to aid in the diagnosis of exocrine pancreatic insufficiency and for differentiating the condition from intestinal malabsorption. A plasma turbidity test can be performed to screen for malabsorption and/or maldigestion of fat. If fat is effectively digested and absorbed, lipemia (plasma turbidity) should be observed within two hours after a fatty meal. The procedure for the plasma turbidity test is outlined in Table 5.

An oral peptide-para-aminobenzoic acid (PABA) digestion test has shown promise as a useful and reliable test for detecting exocrine pancreatic insufficiency. But, it is not yet commercially available.

In the test, a synthetic, chymotrypsin-labile, peptide N-benzoly-L-tyrosyl-para-aminobenzoic acid is given orally to a dog. In normal dogs, the peptide is cleaved by chymotrypsin to yield free PABA, which is subsequently absorbed into the blood and then excreted via the kidneys. The amount of PABA in urine collected for six hours after oral administration of peptide-PABA is used to eval-

TABLE 1—Direct Fecal Microscopy for Detection of Steatorrhea

1. Make a direct smear of fresh feces on two glass slides.

2. Stain one smear with Sudan III and examine it microscopically. The presence of numerous fat globules indicates a positive test. Fat globules will appear as spherical yellow-orange droplets. They indicate that the steatorrhea is caused by maldigestion (undigested neutral fats resulting from an absence of lipase).

3. Mix the second smear with a few drops of acetic acid and Sudan III and heat three times. This procedure converts fatty acids and salts to water-insoluble free fatty acids that will stain with Sudan III.

Fats will appear as orange globules that become sheaths and spicules after cooling. More than 10 globules per high power field indicates steatorrhea. These results indicate malabsorption rather than maldigestion.

TABLE 2—Direct Fecal Microscopy Smears for Detection of Amylorrhea and Creatorrhea

Amylorrhea

Make a direct smear of feces on a glass slide and stain it with Lugol 2% iodine. Examine the smear microscopically. The presence of numerous starch granules indicates a positive test. The granules will appear blue-black with a green birefringence around the edges.

Creatorrhea

Make a direct smear of feces on a glass slide and stain it with New Methylene Blue or clear it with acetic acid. Examine the specimen microscopically. The presence of undigested striated muscle fibers indicates a positive test.

Positive control: Examine a meat-based dog food instead of feces.

TABLE 3—The Gelatin Tube Test (Qualitative Test for Proteolytic Activity (Trypsin) in Feces)

1. Make a 1:10 solution of fecal dilution by adding 1 ml of fresh feces to 9 ml of water. Mix well.

2. Warm three tubes of 7.5% gelatin solution (household gelatin) to 37 C. Add 1 ml of 5% sodium bicarbonate to each tube. To one tube, add 1 ml of feces dilution from the test animal. To the second tube, add 1 ml of water (negative control); and to the third tube, add 1 ml of feces dilution from a normal animal (positive control).

3. Incubate all tubes at 37 C for one hour or at room temperature for two and one-half hours.

4. Refrigerate the tubes for 20 minutes (solidification of the gelatin will occasionally take a little longer). The test is complete when the negative control blank has solidified. Failure of the gelatin to solidify indicates the presence of trypsin in the feces.

TABLE 4—The Radiographic Film Test (Qualitative Test for Proteolytic Activity (Trypsin) in Feces)

1. Make a 1:10 solution of fecal dilution by adding 1 ml of fresh feces to 9 ml of 5% sodium bicarbonate.

2. Place a strip of radiographic film in the fecal dilution. Incubate a second strip of radiographic film in 5% sodium bicarbonate (negative control), and incubate a third strip in a fecal dilution from a normal dog (positive control).

3. Incubate all samples at 37 C for one hour or at room temperature for two and one-half hours.

4. Rinse the film. A clearing of the test film (digestion of the gelatin on the film) where it was soaked with the fecal mixture indicates the presence of trypsin. The negative control should remain unchanged.

uate exocrine pancreatic function. Dogs with exocrine pancreatic insufficiency secrete little chymotrypsin and thus develop a negligible rise in the plasma level of PABA. These animals excrete less than 15% of orally administered PABA in six hours.

Treatment

The basis for treatment of exocrine pancreatic insufficiency is the oral administration of exogenous pancreatic enzymes. The success of enzyme replacement therapy is influenced by 1) the enzyme preparation 2) the schedule of administration, and 3) reducing the gastric degradation of enzymes to improve delivery of active enzyme into the duodenum.

Commercial pancreatic enzyme supplements are extracts of hog or beef pancreas. They are available in powder, tablet, or capsule form and

TABLE 5—Methodology for Plasma-Turbidity or Fat Absorption Test

1. Fast the animal for 12 hours. Then take a presample of plasma and observe for turbidity (lipemia).
2. Administer vegetable oil or Lipomul® (Upjohn) orally at a rate of 3 ml/kg.
3. Take a blood sample at two and three hours after feeding. Compare the plasma with the presample for turbidity.
4. Lack of turbidity suggests malabsorption or maldigestion. In dogs with exocrine pancreatic insufficiency (maldigestion), lack of turbidity is a result of insufficient pancreatic lipase.

The test should then be repeated; pancreatic enzymes (Viokase-V) should be added to the vegetable oil. If this test plasma sample is turbid (lipemic), the diagnosis is exocrine pancreatic insufficiency. If the plasma is not turbid (nonlipemic), the test results indicate malabsorption and additional tests are indicated.

vary in activity and efficacy. Three such products are 1) Viokase-V® (A.H. Robins), which is reliable, reasonably priced and widely used in tablet or powder form; 2) Pancrease® (Johnson & Johnson), which consists of pH-sensitive, enteric-coated microspheres of enzymes; and 3) Cotazym® (Organon), a lipase-enriched, hog pancreas extract.

An effective dosage of Viokase-V is 1 tsp powder/10 lb body weight, or an equivalent amount of crushed Viokase-V tablets, mixed with food. The enzymes and an equivalent volume of sodium bicarbonate should be mixed with food and allowed to incubate 30 to 60 minutes before feeding. This theoretically initiates the digestion process. The animal's daily food intake should be divided into three feedings.

REFERENCES

1. Coffin, D.L.; Thordal-Christensen, A.: The Clinical and Some Pathological Aspects of Pancreatic Disease in the Dog. *Vet. Med.* *48*:193; 1953.
2. Pairent, F.W. *et al*: The Treatment of Pancreatic Exocrine Insufficiency-III. The Effects of Pancreatic Ductal Ligation and Oral Pancreatic Enzyme Supplements on Fecal Lipid Excretion in the Dog. *Ann. Surg.* *170*:737; 1969.
3. Strombeck, D.R.: *Small Animal Gastroenterology.* Stonegate Publishing Company, Davis, Calif., 1979.
4. Anderson, N.V.: Pancreatitis in Dogs. *Vet. Clin. N. Am.* 2:79; 1972.

CHAPTER 25

Laboratory examination

The most important gastric secretory function is the secretion of hydrochloric acid by the gastric parietal cells. Abnormalities include the rarely seen reduction or cessation of acid secretion (achlorhydria) and a relatively common increase in secretion associated with chronic renal disease, chronic hepatic disease, and gastrin-secretory tumors. Acid hypersecretion may be associated with gastric ulcers. Cimetidine (Tagamet® —Smith, Kline, & French) given in doses of 100 to 300 mg three times daily inhibits secretion of hydrochloric acid.

Examination of feces

Fecal examinations should be done for all patients with gastrointestinal problems. The examination should include evaluation of physical qualities (*e.g.* appearance, color, odor) as well as a microscopic examination for parasites and abnormal components (*e.g.* undigested fats, muscle fibers). Occasionally, the feces should be cultured for bacterial pathogens (*e.g. Salmonella* spp and/or *Shigella* spp).

Gross examination

Diarrhea is an increase in the volume or frequency of bowel movements or a change in consistency of feces. Normal feces contain 60 to 70% water; an increase of 10% can produce watery diarrhea. A large volume of normal feces can result from ingestion of excessive amounts of undigestible fiber, which is included in many reducing diets. For a 30-lb dog, the normal volume of formed feces should be approximately 50 ml/24 hours.[1] Normal feces are completely formed; have indentations from colon contractions; and contain no mucus, blood, or undigested food particles.

Normal feces are dark brown because of urobilin, which is produced during metabolism of bilirubin. Excess bilirubin metabolic products, which result from interference with bilirubin metabolism, can cause feces to be orange. In the absence of bilirubin secretions, acholic or gray feces are produced.

Patients with diarrhea always have light-colored feces because of a reduction in numbers of bacteria in the colon. Administration of antibiotics can also produce light-colored feces by reducing numbers of normal intestinal bacteria. Microflora can be suppressed with antibiotics for only a few days.[1]

Black feces are caused by hemorrhage in the upper gastrointestinal tract. Black feces also can be produced by administration of antidiarrheal drugs containing bismuth. Sulfobromophthalein sodium administered to evaluate liver function is excreted in bile and can color feces purple.

Fecal odor is caused by bacterial degradation of tryptophan to indole and skatole compounds and by the metabolism of sulfur-containing amino acids, which produces mercaptans and hydrogen sulfide. Fecal odor is reduced when animals are fed high-carbohydrate diets and increased when high-protein diets are fed. In animals with maldigestion or malabsorption, short-chain fatty acids produced from fermentation of unabsorbed carbohydrates and fatty acids can cause feces to smell acrid.

Microscopic examination

In all cases of diarrhea, feces should be examined microscopically for intestinal parasites and signs of malabsorption or maldigestion. Laboratory techniques for detecting malabsorption and maldigestion have been discussed.[2] Staining fecal smears can aid in identifying leukocytes, which can be present in patients with chronic inflammatory bowel disease.

Evaluation of fecal smears for microorganisms is usually of limited value. The only known intestinal pathogens are *Salmonella* spp and some enteropathic *Escherichia coli*. *Shigella* organisms have been reported only once in dogs, and none of these bacteria can be identified in fecal smears. Spirochetes, part of the normal flora that colonize mucosal crypts and appear in diarrheic feces, are often seen in fecal smears from dogs with diarrhea. Overgrowth of normal intestinal microbes such as *Staphylococcus* spp or *Candida* spp can occur after administration of broad-spectrum antibiotics.

Microscopic examination of feces for parasites involves flotation and sedimentation tests. Most parasites are easily identified microscopically by their ova. There are excellent texts containing photomicrographs of parasitic ova and parasites.[3,4]

Tapeworms pass proglottids in the stool, and these are usually noticed by owners. Tapeworm ova will not be visible microscopically unless the packets containing the ova are ruptured. Multiple fecal examinations may be necessary to diagnose whipworms. Protozoan parasites such as *Giardia* spp and *Trichomonas* spp are often difficult to identify and are usually most easily diagnosed in fresh stool. The living parasites are best observed in direct smears made from feces diluted with normal saline solution.

Parasite ova are easier to find if feces are concentrated before microscopic examination. For concentration, feces are mixed in a saturated solution of zinc sulfate, magnesium sulfate, salt, or sugar. Flotation is done after a suspension of feces has stood in the solution. Ova adhere to a glass slide or coverslip placed in contact with the top of the solution. Flotation can be hastened by centrifuging the suspension and placing a drop from the surface of the solution onto a glass slide.

Fluke ova are concentrated by sedimentation. Feces are mixed with water, and the solution is strained through gauze and centrifuged. Next, the supernatant is poured off and the sediment examined microscopically.

Miscellaneous tests

Occult blood

Feces may contain small amounts of blood not visible grossly (occult blood). Bleeding from the gastrointestinal tract can be detected with chemical tests based on blood peroxidase activity. Rapid and sensitive tests for occult blood are Occultest (Ames) and Hemoccult (Smith, Kline & French). The tests are so sensitive that to avoid false positives, animals should not be fed meat for three days before testing.

Total fecal fat

Determination of total fecal fat aids in detecting steatorrhea. A standard diet with a known quantity of fat is fed for several days before collection of feces. Next, feces are collected for 24 hours and mixed with a small amount of water. The mixture is homogenized, and the amount of fat in a representative aliquot is determined. In normal dogs, less than 5% of total dietary fat remains in the feces. Quantitation of fecal fat does not provide a diagnosis but indicates the presence of steatorrhea.

Digestion and absorption test

The procedure for performing lipid-absorption tests and the interpretation of these tests have been discussed.[2]

The D-xylose absorption test provides the easiest means of identifying malabsorption. Xylose is a five-carbon monosaccharide that is absorbed passively from the jejunum into the portal circulation. Its absorption does not require the lymphatic system or any special transport mechanism. Variables that affect absorption of D-xylose include 1) the amount administered, 2) the rate of gastric emptying, 3) the mucosal surface area of the small bowel, and 4) the intestinal blood circulation.

The amount of xylose administered is based on body weight. Delayed gastric emptying should be ruled out by radiography before absorption tests are done, thus leaving only two variables: intestinal mucosal surface area and intestinal blood circulation. D-xylose (500 mg/kg) is given as a 10 to 25% solution via stomach tube to the fasted patient. The tube is flushed with water after administration. Blood samples for xylose determinations are obtained before administration and at 0.5, 1, 2, 3, 4, and 5 hours afterwards.

The most accurate results are obtained when samples are sent to a commercial laboratory for evaluation. If any value is above 50 mg/dl, then the jejunal absorption for pentoses is normal. If none of the values exceeds 50 mg/dl, then malabsorption is present or intestinal circulation is impaired. The most common causes of malabsorption are 1) reduction of mucosal surface area by atrophy of the villi, or 2) cellular infiltration, which occurs in cases of eosinophilic gastroenterocolitis. Lymphangiectasia has no effect on the absorption of xylose. When results of the D-xylose absorption test indicate malabsorption, a biopsy is required for a definitive diagnosis. In some cases, evaluation with hypoallergenic, gluten-free diets (d/d—Hills) or low-fat, gluten-free diets (i/d—Hills) is necessary.

REFERENCES

1. Strombeck, D.R.: Small Animal Gastroenterology. Stonegate Publishing, Davis, California, 1979.
2. Seybold, I.M. *et al*: Practitioners Laboratory II—Exocrine Pancreatis-2. *VM/SAC* 76:1709-1711; 1981.
3. Sloss, M. *et al*: *Veterinary Clinical Parasitology*, 5th ed. Iowa State University Press, Ames, Iowa, 1978.
4. Williams, J.F.; Zajac, A.: Diagnosis of Gastrointestinal Parasitism in Dogs and Cats. Ralston Purina, St. Louis, Mo., 1980.

CHAPTER 26

Management of gastrointestinal problems

MANY GASTROINTESTINAL diseases cause disruption of the patient's fluid, electrolyte, and nutrient balances. Fluid and electrolyte imbalances, usually associated with acute diseases of the gastrointestinal tract, can create critical situations requiring immediate clinical action. Nutrient imbalances are associated with chronic diseases of the gastrointestinal tract and seldom require emergency treatment. Recovery from nutrient imbalance in best achieved with sound dietary management rather than through use of drugs. Often the primary reason for treating a chronic gastrointestinal problem is the nuisance of uncontrolled elimination of feces.

Fluid and electrolyte balance

Gastrointestinal problems cause fluid and electrolyte imbalances primarily through a loss of water and electrolytes, which results from vomiting and/or diarrhea. The body can usually compensate for the loss of sodium. However, the potassium level in gastrointestinal secretions is at least twice the plasma level, resulting in a disproportionate loss of potassium. The loss of potassium from the gastrointestinal tract is not compensated for by the body and thus, potassium should be added when the intravascular fluid balance is corrected.

Recommended intravenous replacement fluids for vomiting patients are Ringer solution (without lactate) or 0.9% sodium chloride. Forty milliequivalents of potassium chloride solution can be added to a liter of balanced Ringer solution to make a 44 mEq/L concentration of potassium, or to a liter of balanced sodium chloride solution to make a 40 mEq/L concentration of potassium. These solutions should be given at a rate not to exceed 0.25 mEq of potassium/lb/hour. The total amount of potassium to be given can be determined by monitoring an electrocardiogram or measuring serum potassium levels. Additional intravenous fluids (without the potassium supplement) can be given as needed.

To treat animals with diarrhea, lactated Ringer solution or other balanced electrolyte solutions can be used initially without supplemental potassium. If anorexia and/or diarrhea continue for several days, supplementation of potassium as described above may be needed. (See explanation box below for method of calculating required dose of intravenous fluids.)

Pharmaceuticals

Drugs are often overused in the treatment of gastrointestinal disease. The most important treatment

Here's how to calculate the required dose of intravenous fluids ▶

for gastrointestinal problems is rest of the gastrointestinal tract. For acute problems, this is accomplished by restricting oral intake of food and water. When complete restriction of food and water is required for longer periods, nutrients and fluids can be administered parenterally.

Patients with acute gastritis and emesis often require antiemetics and antibacterial drugs. Among the most effective antiemetics are the phenothiazine tranquilizers, which exhibit antiemetic activity at a fraction of the dose necessary to produce tranquilization. One of the most effective of these drugs is Thorazine® (SmithKline & French). Antihistamines such as dimenhydrinate and meclizine are also used, but are primarily for the control of motion sickness. Gastric acid secretion can be reduced with histamine analogs such as cimetidine (Tagamet® —SmithKline & French) given at a dose of 100 to 300 mg three times daily, or the gastric acid can be neutralized with antacids. However, if renal perfusion is inadequate, neutralization with antacids such as sodium bicarbonate can result in alkalosis. Milk is not an antacid and should not be used to treat acute gastritis.

The amount of intravenous fluids given depends on the estimated degree of dehydration. The total fluid deficit can be calculated from this formula: **(percent dehydration) × (body weight in pounds) × (500 ml) = total body fluid deficit in milliliters.** *This amount added to the amount of normal daily loss (usually about 25 to 30 ml/lb) should be given over a 24-hour period. Subsequent fluid replacement can be calculated as the normal daily loss (25 to 30 ml/lb) added to any extra loss (e.g. vomitus) that can be estimated.*

Antibiotics are seldom necessary for the treatment of gastrointestinal disease. Procaine penicillin G given intramuscularly once daily at a dose of 20,000 units/lb is the most effective treatment against anaerobes, kanamycin (Kantrim® —Bristol) given subcutaneously twice daily at a dose of 2.5 mg/lb is effective against aerobes. Orally administered nonabsorbable antibiotics such as neomycin are of no value.[1] The goal of antibiotic therapy is prevention of systemic bacterial invasion, not sterilization of the gastrointestinal mucosa.

Modifiers of gut motility should usually be avoided. Anticholinergics such as atropine and scopolamine reduce motility by inhibiting peristalsis, but can also cause paralytic ileus. Reduction of motility increases the time allowed for bacteria to multiply and invade other tissues. Modifiers of motility that stimulate rhythmic segmentation (Lomotil® —Searle) given at a child's dosage may be beneficial to treat common diarrhea but are contraindicated for treating acute hemorrhagic diarrhea.

Intestinal protectants such as kaolin, pectin, bismuth subsalicylate, and magnesium trisilicate are of some benefit in absorbing bacteria and toxins. However, except when given in massive doses, they are probably ineffective for coating the inflamed mucosa. The recommended dose of Kaopectate® (Upjohn) is 1 oz/10 lb given every two to four hours, and for bismuth subsalicylate is 2 ml/lb given every six hours. (Bismuth can cause black feces. This should not be interpreted as hemorrhage from the gastrointestinal tract.) Few gastrointestinal disorders are responsive to long-term pharmacologic therapy. Notable exceptions are eosinophilic gastroenterocolitis, which is responsive to corticosteroids, and chronic colitis, which is responsive to Azulfidine® (Pharmacia) given at a dose of 30 mg/

lb three times daily. The total daily dose should not exceed 3 grams. Because Azulfidine is broken down in the colon into a sulfa derivative and an aspirin derivative, it should not be given to cats.

Diet

Dietary management is the most important aspect of treating chronic gastrointestinal disorders. An ideal diet for patients with gastrointestinal disorders requires little or no digestion, contains little fat, is free of lactose and gluten, and is hypoallergenic and palatable. When the absorptive capacity of the intestinal tract is compromised, fats are the first nutrients to escape absorption. Excessive fat reaching the colon is an irritant that intensifies diarrhea. The medium- and short-chain fatty acids are sometimes used in diets because they are water soluble, more readily absorbed, and do not require lymphatic transport as do regular fats. Lactose should be eliminated from the diet because lactase is deficient in all patients with diarrhea.[2] Osmotic diarrhea results from bacterial degradation of undigested lactose reaching the colon.

Commercial and prescription diets are available for some types of gastrointestinal disorders. The Prescription Diet d/d® (Hills) is made from mutton and rice. It is gluten-free, palatable, and hypoallergenic. The new formula for Prescription Diet i/d® (Hills) contains cottage cheese, egg, rice, liver, corn grits, corn starch, animal fat, soy grits, and sugar. It is palatable, low fat, and gluten-free. Commercial diets that are best for patients with gastrointestinal disorders are Science maximum-stress diet, IAMS chunks, and IAMS Eukanuba.[1] The Prescription Diets c/d® and p/d® (Hills) are useful for cats with diarrhea.

Elemental diets are available as supportive nutrition for anorectic animals. These liquid, low-volume diets contain high levels of protein and carbohydrates but only medium-chain triglycerides. Isocal Portagen® and Sustacal® (Mead Johnson) are used to maintain nutrition in debilitated anorectic animals with gastrointestinal disease. These diets can be fed via stomach tube or other force-feeding methods.

Total parenteral nutrition is sometimes needed to completely rest the gastrointestinal tract and simultaneously maintain a relative nutritional balance. A mixture of 350 ml Intralipid® (Cutter), 100 ml of 10% dextrose, and 100 ml of 8% Travasol® (Cutter) given intravenously over a 24-hour period provides total parenteral nutrition for one day for a 25-lb dog. This suspension should be given via a long intravenous catheter (Intracath® —Abott) in a volume not to exceed 22 ml/lb/day.

REFERENCES

1. Strombeck, D.R.: *Small Animal Gastroenterology*. Stonegate Publishing, Davis, Calif., 1979.
2. Newcomer, A.D.; Disaccharidase Deficiencies. *Mayo Clin. Proc.* *48*:648-652; 1973.

CHAPTER 27

A systematic approach to obtaining an electrocardiograph

ELECTROCARDIOLOGY is a diagnostic tool for evaluating the heart. An electrocardiogram (ECG) is a quick, easy method of measuring cardiac changes and differentiating arrhythmias. It is also used to assess the efficacy of cardiac therapy (*e.g.* digitalis, quinidine) and to evaluate traumatic patients, metabolic problems (*e.g.* eclampsia, electrolyte imbalance, ketoacidosis), patients with epilepsy, and the presence of toxins. In anesthetized patients, the T wave, heart rate, S-T segment, and arrhythmias are observed when the depth of anesthesia is monitored. Serial ECGs are helpful for following the progression of premature ventricular contractions, atrioventricular block, and atrial fibrillation. Electrocardiograms are a routine part of presurgical examinations and are commonly used as a means of preventive medicine for older patients.

For both dogs and cats, the ECG is usually taken with the animal in right lateral recumbency; the limbs should be perpendicular to the body and parallel to one another. Electrocardiograms of the feline heart may also be taken while the animal is in sternal recumbency. A quiet room should be reserved for recording ECGs, and the ECG machine should be kept in a permanent location. This permits standardization of the machine and reduces artifacts. Procedures for correcting artifacts are shown in Table 1. The ECG should be placed in a folder and included in the animal's permanent file.

Paper speed is set at 50 mm/second. At this speed, each horizontal square on the paper equals 0.02 seconds. Ten vertical squares equal 1 millivolt (mv). Electrodes are placed on each limb at the stifles and elbows, and/or other areas of the body. A strip of paper 6 to 12 inches long is run on each lead. Leads are listed in Table 2.

The heart acts as a functional syncytium in that any area of the heart that discharges electrical activity continues to spread this activity throughout the heart. As electrical activity spreads, the cardiac muscle contracts. The usual pathway of these electrical impulses is the sinoatrial node (located within the right atria), atrioventricular node, junctional tissue, bundle of His, bundle fibers, Purkinje fibers, and finally, dorsally from the tip of the ventricles. Because the sinoatrial node normally depolarizes first, it is known as the pacemaker.

The ECG complex includes P, Q, R, S, and T waves. Also, measurements are taken of the P-R interval and segment, the S-T segment, and the Q-T interval. The various waves represent:

1. *P waves* — atrial depolarization or contraction.
2. *Q waves* — depolarization of the ventricular septum.
3. *R waves* — depolarization of the ventricles.
4. *S waves* — depolarization of the base of the ventricles.
5. *T waves* — repolarization of the ventricles.

The QRS complex represents the total depolarization time of the heart. The P-R interval is the time required for an impulse to travel from the sinoatrial node to the ventricles. The P-R segment is the time it takes an impulse to reach the atrioventricular node. The S-T segment indicates ventricular repo-

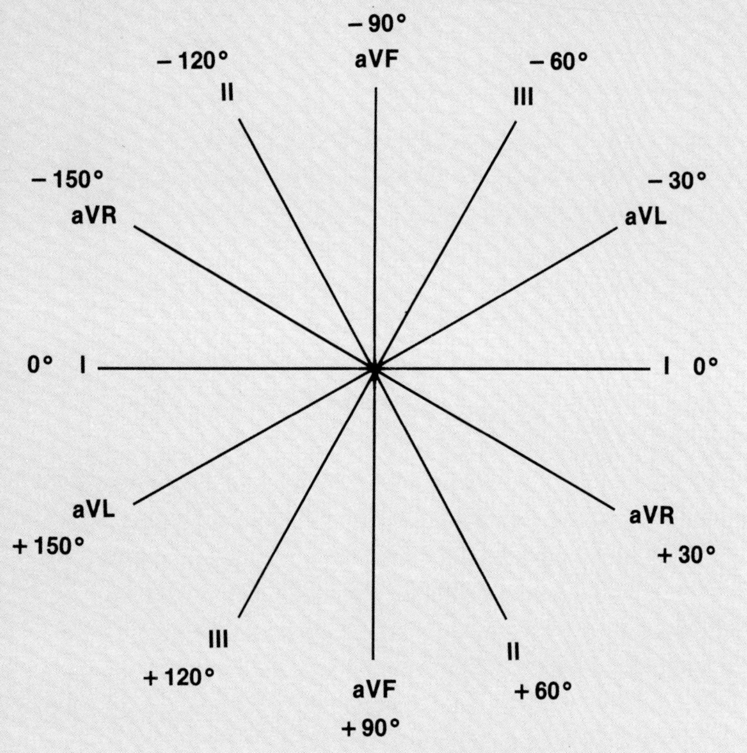

Figure 1—Bailey's six axis reference system.

larization. Changes in these parameters signal possible abnormalities in the area of the heart represented by each parameter.

Systematic approach to electrocardiography

A systematic approach to recording an ECG includes evaluation of the heart rate, cardiac rhythm, mean electrical axis (MEA), parameters, and of miscellaneous criteria (including arrhythmias).

Heart rate and rhythm

All measurements are taken from Lead II, unless otherwise indicated. The heart rate is determined by counting the R waves between three of the small vertical marks at the top of the ECG paper. (When the paper speed is 50 mm/sec., the space between two of these marks equals 1.5 seconds). The number of R waves between three marks multiplied by 20 equals the heart rate in beats/minute. Normal heart rate for dogs ranges from 60 to 160 beats/min., depending on size. Feline heart rates average 140 to 240 beats/minute.

The heart rate is measured to check rhythm. A gross overview of the ECG is examined and R-R intervals are compared. If they are not the same, then an arrhythmia is present. Sinus rhythm is defined as a P wave for each QRS complex and a QRS complex for each P wave. Three rhythms are normal for dogs: 1) normal sinus rhythm, 2) sinus arrhythmia, and 3) wandering pacemaker. If each R-R interval is the same, then sinus rhythm is present. In animals with sinus arrhythmia, variability among R-R intervals exists. A wandering pacemaker is evidenced by varying voltages of the P wave, an indication that several areas close to the normal pacemaker are acting as the pacemaker. In evaluating rhythm, all P waves and QRS complexes are examined for similar configurations and relationships.

Mean electrical axis

The MEA is a measurement of the mean electrical activity (cardiac vector) of the heart when the ventricles depolarize. Direction of the force of electrical activity is determined by evaluating the QRS complexes in each of the six leads of Bailey's hexaxial system (*Figure 1*). Normal MEA for dogs is between +40 degrees and +100 degrees.[1] If the axis shifts toward the left limb or is less than +40 degrees, left axis deviation is recorded, indicating hypertrophy of the left ventricle. Left axis shift is between +40 degrees and −90 degrees, though a shift of more than 60 degrees is rare. Shifts greater than +100 degrees indicate right axis deviation and suggest hypertrophy of the right ventricle. If both ventricles are enlarged, the axis remains normal.

The vector can be calculated mathematically but the following procedure is adequate for determining the mean electrical axis.

1. Find the isoelectical lead, *i.e.* lead that has as much negative deflection as positive deflection or is as close to a straight line as possible.

2. Use a six-axis reference chart (*Figure 1*) to determine which lead is perpendicular to the isoelectric lead.

3. Determine whether the perpendicular lead is positive or negative (positive or negative deflection of the QRS complex).

If a positive deflection occurs, then the electrical impulse is traveling toward the positive pole of

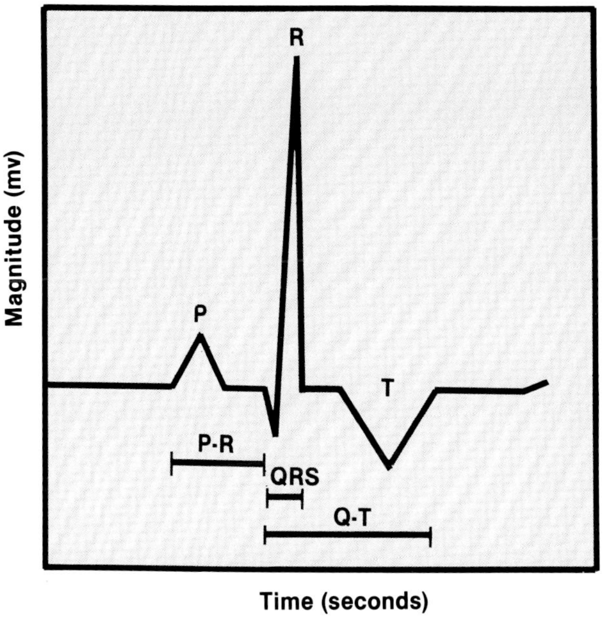

Figure 2—Normal measurements for ECG parameters:
P wave: From beginning to end of P wave and from top to bottom.
P-R interval: From beginning of P wave to beginning of QRS complex.
QRS complex: From beginning to end of QRS complex and from baseline to top of R wave.
S-T segment: Between end of S wave to beginning of T wave. Runs along the baseline before going into the T wave.
T wave: Measure from baseline to apex.
Q-T interval: From beginning of Q wave to end of T wave.

TABLE 1—Correction of Artifacts

1. Clips should be clean and tightly attached to the cables. Use sandpaper to remove rust or corrosion, or replace clips.
2. Firmly attach leads to animal. Check to see that skin contact is good. Use some alcohol to wet leads, but not so much that electrical contact is established between two clips. Keep the tabletop dry.
3. Do not allow clips to touch one another.
4. The person holding the animal should not touch any clips.
5. Check the ground cord. Improper grounding will interfere with proper electrical conduction, producing 60-cycle interference.
6. If the machine has a ground switch, flip it back and forth until a setting is reached that produces a smooth, steady tracing.
7. Turn out room lights (especially fluorescent lights).
8. Place animal on a rubber mat or wool blanket for insulation.
9. Unplug any electrical appliances on the same circuit as the machine.
10. Try procedure using a different animal holder.
11. Remove any electric watches from the vicinity. Not only can the watch cause an artifact, but the machine can cause the watch to malfunction.
12. Move equipment and animal to a different room or area and review this checklist if interference continues.

the lead. If two leads are isoelectric, either may be used. However, if all leads are isoelectric, the term *electrically vertical heart* is used, and the MEA cannot be determined.

Parameters

Heights and widths of the P wave, P-R interval, QRS complex, R wave, S-T segment, T wave, and Q-T segment should be obtained (*Figure 2*).

The P wave, the first positive deflection preceding the QRS complex, indicates atrial depolarization and contraction. It is used to measure the size of both atria. Normal parameters are given in Table 3. A P wave taller than 0.4 mv is known as P pulmonale and indicates hypertrophy of the right atrium. Depression of the P-R segment indicates hypertrophy of the right atrium. P mitrale, a P wave greater than 0.04 sec., indicates hypertrophy of the left atrium. A notched P wave with normal measurements is not abnormal.

The P-R interval is measured from beginning of the P wave to beginning of the QRS complex. The normal P-R interval for dogs is 0.06-0.13 seconds. The P-R interval is prolonged 0.02-0.03 sec. when an animal is given digitalis. First-degree heart block is evidenced by a P-R interval exceeding 0.13 seconds. If the P-R interval varies from QRS complex to QRS complex, a cardiac arrhythmia is present. The P-R interval varies inversely to the heart rate.

Deep voltage (greater than 0.5 mv) Q waves are

an indication of right ventricular hypertrophy; the Q wave is the first negative deflection after the P wave. The QRS complex is measured from beginning of the Q wave to end of the S wave. Left ventricular hypertrophy is indicated by a wide and tall QRS complex with a slurred S-T segment. A QRS complex greater than 0.7 sec. in duration can indicate a bundle branch block. Other ECG parameters should be examined to differentiate this lesion from ventricular enlargement. The S-T segment is measured from the end of the S wave to the beginning of the T wave. It is abnormal for this segment to be elevated or depressed from the baseline. Depression of the S-T segment may indicate left ventricular hypertrophy, myocarditis, hypoxia, or hypercalcemia. Elevation of the S-T segment is seen in patients with myocardial hypoxia, myocarditis, and hypercalcemia.

A normal T wave is positive (40%), negative (60%) or isoelectric in dogs. The T wave is negative in lead V_{10} (except in Chihuahuas) but is positive in patients with heartworm disease. Voltage should be no larger than one-fourth of the R-wave. If the T wave reverses polarity, myocardial hypoxia is occurring. Tall spiked T waves indicate hyperkalemia; small biphasic waves indicate hypokalemia.

Q-T intervals (normally 0.14 to 0.22 sec. long) are measured from beginning of the Q wave to end of the T wave. Like the P-R interval, the Q-T interval varies inversely with the heart rate. The concentration of certain electrolytes alters the Q-T interval. Hypokalemia, or hypocalcemia may prolong the Q-T interval, and hyperkalemia may either shorten or prolong the Q-T interval.

TABLE 2—Electrocardiography Leads

Bailey's Hexaxial Leads
Lead I
Lead II
Lead III

Augmented Unipolar Leads
Augmented vector right (aVR)
Augmented vector left (aVL)
Augmented vector feet (aVF)

Orthogonal Leads
x (equal to lead I)
y (equal to lead aVF)
z (equal to lead V_{10})

Esophageal

Percordial (Unipolar)
CV_6LL — left sixth intercostal space at sternum
CV_6LU — left sixth intercostal space at costochondral junction
CV_5RL — right fifth intercostal space at sternum
V_{10} — over the seventh thoracic vertebra

Miscellaneous parameters

Right ventricular hypertrophy or septal hypertrophy is indicated by deep voltage Q waves in Leads II, III, and aVF; deep S waves in CV_6LR; and positive T waves in V_{10}. Deep voltage Q waves greater than 0.5 mv suggest hypertrophy of the right ventricle. The S wave in CV_6LU should be greater than 0.7 mv before it is considered indicative of right ventricular hypertrophy. Right ventricular enlargement is considered present when the MEA is between +100 degrees and −90 degrees. When both ventricles are enlarged, the MEA is usually normal, the S-T segment is slurred, the P wave is tall and/or wide, the QRS complex is wide, and the R wave is tall (greater than 2.5 mv).

Mild hyperkalemia (6.0 to 6.5 mEq/liter) causes T waves to become tall and peaked, but the P wave and QRS complex remain normal. When the potassium concentration increases to 6.5 to 7.0 mEq/liter, the heart rate slows, P waves flatten, and T waves continue to be tall. High potassium levels (greater than 7.5 mEq/liter) cause the heart rate to slow to less than 60 beats/min. (atrial standstill) and cause a prolonged Q-T interval and possible increased voltage of T waves. Potassium levels greater than 9.5 mEq/liter cause cardiac arrest. In patients with renal insufficiency, hyperkalemia may result in complete heart block. Hydrocortisone, dextrose in saline solution, and desoxycorticosterone acetate

TABLE 3—Normal Values for Electrocardiogram Measurements

	Dogs	Cats
Heart		
Rates	60-160 beats/min. in adults Up to 180 beats/min. in toy breeds	240 beats/min. maximum
Parameters		
P Wave	Width: Max. 0.04 sec. Height: 0.04 mv	Positive in leads II and AVF; may be isoelectric or positive in lead I; should not exceed 0.04 sec. in duration
P-R interval	Width: 0.06 to 0.13 sec.	0.04 to 0.10 sec. duration
QRS complex	Width: Max. 0.05 sec. — toy breeds Max. 0.06 sec. — large breeds	The mean electrical axis in the frontal plane is often insignificant. Often the QRS complex is nearly isoelectric in all frontal plane limb leads Duration — Less than 0.04 sec.
R wave	Height: Max. 2.5 mv — toy breeds Max. 3.0 mv — larger breeds	Usually low in amplitude. R wave over 1.0 mv in the frontal plane leads suggests ventricular hypertrophy

	Dogs	Cats
Rhythms	Normal sinus rhythms Sinus arrhythmia Wandering pacemaker	Normal sinus rhythm Sinus arrhythmia (infrequently)
Axis	$+40^{\circ}$ to $+100^{\circ}$ $+40^{\circ}$ to $+90^{\circ}$ in toy breeds	0° to $+100^{\circ}$
S-T segment	No S-T depression Should not lie more than 0.2 mv below baseline in lead II; Not depressed more than 0.1 to 0.2 mv in lead III No S-T elevation Should not lie more than 0.15 mv above the baseline in lead II or III	Should be small and free of repolarization changes, marked depression, or marked elevation.
T Wave	Can be positive or negative or biphasic in most leads. Should be negative in lead V_{10} (except Chihuahuas). Generally not higher than ¼ of the amplitude of the R wave.	Should be small and free of repolarization changes, marked depression, or marked elevation.
Q-T interval	Width: 0.14 sec. to 0.22 sec. Varies with heart rate; slower heart rates have longer Q-T intervals.	

(DOCA) may be used to treat this block.

Hypokalemia (3.0 mEq/liter or less) occurs less frequently than does hyperkalemia. Common causes of hypokalemia are excessive use of diuretics, severe vomiting, and diarrhea. The condition is indicated by bradycardia, prolonged Q-T interval, and small biphasic T waves on the ECG. Potassium levels lower than 2.0 mEq/liter are very serious.

Hypocalcemia seldom occurs in animals. When it does, ECG signs are similar to those seen in patients with hypokalemia: the heart rate slows and the Q-T interval is prolonged. Hypercalcemia primarily results in an elevated S-T segment.

Arrhythmias frequently occur in animals, and the only way to differentiate them is with an ECG.

REFERENCE

1. Bolton, G.R.: *Handbook of Canine Electrocardiography*. W. B. Saunders, Philadelphia, Pa., 1975.

CHAPTER 28

Supraventricular arrhythmias

An arrhythmia can only be identified by means of electrocardiography. Arrhythmias have many metabolic, traumatic, congenital, toxic, and primary cardiac causes. Three primary factors should be considered when determining whether an arrhythmia is abnormal: 1) association with respiration, 2) similarity of heart rate and femoral pulse, and 3) presence of a jugular pulse. Because it is important to classify arrhythmias, the classifications are listed in Tables 1 and 2. Arrhythmias are commonly labeled *supraventricular* or *ventricular*.

General considerations

Arrhythmias are evaluated by examining parameters on Lead II. First, it should be determined whether the heart rate is normal or abnormal. Next, heart rhythm should be checked by comparing R-R intervals. Determining whether there is a P wave for each QRS complex and vice versa reveals whether the rhythm is sinus in origin. Also, the P-R intervals should be constant. All P waves should have similar configurations, as should all QRS complexes. If these parameters are different, ectopic foci are discharging intermittently.

Normal sinus rhythm, sinus arrhythmia, and wandering pacemaker are all considered normal. Respiration influences the tone of the vagus nerve, thus increasing and decreasing the heart rate. Inhalation elevates the heart rate, causing it to be regularly irregular, which is sinus arrhythmia.

Normal sinus rhythm is indicated by equal R-R intervals. For cases of sinus arrhythmia R-R intervals vary up to twice as long as normal, whereas for cases of sinus arrest, certain R-R intervals are at least twice as long as normal. If the voltage of the P wave varies, the patient has a wandering pacemaker. In such cases, the P wave may become negative.

Sinus arrest may cause bradycardia, which may result in syncope during exercise. Cervical or thoracic masses can exert pressure on the vagus nerve and cause syncope. Vagal arrhythmias usually respond to treatment with atropine. In cases of vagal arrhythmias the heart rate is normal, there are no pulse deficits, heart rhythm is regularly irregular and of sinus origin, and P-R intervals are constant.

Most pathologic arrhythmias are classified as supraventricular or ventricular. Supraventricular arrhythmias are subdivided into atrial and nodal. But, it is not important to differentiate them because both are treated similarly. Abnormal P waves and normal QRS complexes indicate a supraventricular arrhythmia. A ventricular arrhythmia is evidenced by abnormal QRS complexes, varying P-R intervals, and a possible lack of P waves.

Supraventricular arrhythmias

Supraventricular arrhythmias are most commonly associated with atrioventricular valvular insufficiency. Tumors, toxemias, and digitalis intoxication are other causes. Patients with supraventricular arrhythmias usually have severe mitral insufficiency with congestive heart failure. These arrhythmias are generally treated with digitalis.

Sinus tachycardia

Sinus tachycardia is the most common arrhythmia in dogs. Although it is usually caused by nervousness, it can be initiated by congestive heart failure, pneumonia, fever, anemia, shock, or hyperthyroidism. Signs of sinus tachycardia include a heart rate greater than 160 beats/min (180 beats/min in toy breeds), a regularly irregular heart rhythm of sinus origin, and constant P-R intervals. Sinus tachycardia is differentiated from atrial tachycardia (a more serious arrhythmia) by the P waves. In cases of sinus tachycardia, the P waves are always the same whether the heart rate is normal or tachycardia is occurring. Therapy usually involves treating the primary disease.

Sinus bradycardia

Sinus bradycardia is uncommon in dogs or cats. It is indicated by a heart rate of less than 70 beats/min (dogs) and no pulse deficit or jugular pulse. The primary clinical sign of this condition is weakness. Hyperkalemia, tranquilizers, and sedatives are possible causes. If treatment is required, atropine or isoproterenol is the drug of choice.

Premature contractions

Atrial or junctional premature contractions are evidenced by a normal heart rate, an irregular rhythm with pauses after premature contractions, similar P-R intervals, alterations in the P waves of premature beats, and normal QRS complexes. The P wave may be hidden in the T wave during the premature contractions.

Atrial tachycardia

Atrial tachycardia is a serious arrhythmia that resembles sinus tachycardia on an ECG. However, in cases of atrial tachycardia, the tachycardia usually occurs in bursts with possible atrial premature beats. Continuous tachycardia indicates sinus tachycardia. Placing digital pressure on the eyes or at the bifurcation of the carotid arteries increases the tone of the vagus nerve, thus ending atrial tachycardia. The same technique has little or no effect on sinus tachycardia.

TABLE 1—Classification of Arrhythmias[1]

Classification with Regard to Therapy

Supraventricular
- Sinus bradycardia
- Sinus tachycardia
- Wandering pacemaker
- Sinus arrhythmia
- Sinus arrest
- Sinoatrial block
- Atrial flutter
- Atrial tachycardia
- Atrial fibrillation
- Junctional tachycardia
- Atrial premature contractions

Ventricular
- Premature ventricular contractions
- Ventricular tachycardia
- Ventricular fibrillation
- Atrioventricular dissociation

Escape Beats
- Junctional escape beats
- Ventricular escape beats

Classification by Heart Rate

Tachycardia
- Sinus tachycardia
- Atrial flutter
- Atrial tachycardia
- Atrial fibrillation
- Junctional tachycardia
- Ventricular tachycardia

Bradycardia
- Sinus bradycardia
- Sinus arrest
- Sinoatrial standstill
- Ventricular escape rhythms
- Junctional escape rhythms
- Complete heart block
- Certain secondary heart block

TABLE 2—Cardiac Arrhythmias Associated with Normal Heart Rates[1]

- Sinus arrhythmia
- Sinus arrest (some)
- Atrial premature beats
- Junctional premature beats
- Ventricular premature beats
- Junctional tachycardia (some)
- Ventricular tachycardia (some)
- Primary heart block
- Secondary heart block
- Bundle branch block
- Wolff - Parkinson - White (W-P-W) Syndrome

Atrial tachycardia is more serious than atrial premature contractions and occurs in conjunction with severe mitral insufficiency, aortic body tumors, and congestive heart failure. Pulse deficits may be present, but no jugular pulse is noted. Weakness, lethargy, ataxia, and intermittent syncope are frequent clinical signs. Seizures may occur.

Atrial tachycardia is seen most often in older animals with severe mitral insufficiency. The ECG shows intermittent tachycardia, constant R-R intervals, sinus origin, constant P-R intervals, and normal QRS complexes. During tachycardia, the P waves are positive but different than they are when the heart rate is normal.

Digitalis is most commonly used to treat this condition. Vasopressors such as phenylephrine and methoxamine are used but care should be exercised when using them to treat patients suffering from congestive heart failure.

Atrial flutter

Atrial flutter is rare in dogs and cats and indicates severe atrial disease. On an ECG tracing, it appears similar to atrial tachycardia. The ECG indicates a normal to rapid heart rate, regular to irregular heart rhythm, no P-R intervals, normal QRS complexes, and P waves replaced by fibrillating waves (f waves). Digitalis is used initially to treat the condition. Subsequently, quinidine is used in an attempt to convert the arrhythmia to normal.

Atrial fibrillation

Atrial fibrillation, which commonly occurs in large to giant breeds of dogs, is also an indication of severe atrial disease. A severe atrioventricular valvular insufficiency usually causes atrial enlargement, resulting in atrial fibrillation. Usually, by the time this abnormality develops, the prognosis is grave. Biventricular congestive heart failure, primary myocardial disease, and congestive cardiomyopathies are routinely associated with atrial fibrillation.

Intolerance for exercise, ascites, coughing, and dyspnea are common clinical signs. Also, the patient's history may include nonresponsive soft stools or diarrhea. Mitral insufficiency, idiopathic cardiomyopathy, patent ductus arteriosis, ventricular septal defects, and pulmonic stenosis are some of the diseases found in conjunction with atrial fibrillation. Rarely, animals with atrial fibrillation may be asymptomatic.

Atrial fibrillation is evidenced by a rapid, irregular heart rate of greater than 160/beats/min, f waves, and normal QRS complexes. The f waves are small undulations of the base line that replace P waves. A jugular pulse, pulse deficit, and a gallop rhythm (third heart beat) may be present.

Initially, the treatment of choice is digitalis to slow the heart rate. Also, diuretics and aminophylline are administered, and salt intake and exercise are restricted. As the heart rate is reduced and the congestive heart failure controlled, quinidine can be given in an effort to convert the fibrillatory pattern to normal sinus rhythm. However, this is usually unsuccessful. (DC cardioversion has been used to achieve temporary conversion to sinus rhythm.) Most patients live only four to six months after atrial fibrillation is diagnosed.

Junctional tachycardia

Junctional (nodal) tachycardia most often results from digitalis intoxication. Severe atrioventricular valvular insufficiency and vagal hypertonicity (inflammation) may cause the condition. Weakness, lethargy, and syncope are common clinical signs. The heart rate is normal to tachycardia with a regular rhythm. The P waves are negative, and the QRS complexes are positive. Digitalis is used to treat junctional tachycardia, unless a toxicity is present from digitalis.

REFERENCE

1. Bolton, R.G.: *Handbook of Canine ECG.* W.B. Saunders, Philadelphia, Pa., 1975.

CHAPTER 29

Ventricular arrhythmias

PRIMARY VENTRICULAR arrhythmias are uncommon in small animals. Generally, they occur secondarily to viral, bacterial, mycotic, protozoan, or parasitic pericarditis; digitalis treatment; mitral insufficiencies; hypoxia; acidosis; cardiomyopathies; diabetes mellitus; or hypo- or hyperthyroidism. These abnormalities cause myocardial irritation, which results in premature ventricular contractions (PVC) and ventricular tachycardia.

Abnormal clinical signs are seldom seen when PVC occur at a rate of not more than one every five minutes. But, when PVC become more frequent, weakness, intolerance to exercise, collapse, coma, seizures, or sudden death may occur. Pulse deficits are found in patients with PVC and ventricular tachycardia. A jugular pulse may also be present.

Electrocardiographic signs of PVC include a normal heart rate but an irregular rhythm. Also, P-R intervals are abnormal, and the P wave is unrelated to the premature and bizarre QRS complex. (Normal QRS complexes are related to P waves.) The configuration of the QRS complex indicates whether the PVC are similar and unifocal or unsimilar and multifocal, revealing whether the myocardial irritation is in one or several areas.

Premature ventricular contractions occur singularly, in pairs, or in a run of three. If every other beat is a PVC, this is known as ventricular bigeminy. Ventricular trigeminy is present if every third beat is a PVC. Four or more consecutive PVC indicate ventricular tachycardia.

Also diagnostic of ventricular tachycardia are fusion and/or capture beats. Capture beats are normal beats that interrupt ventricular tachycardia. A fusion beat occurs when normal electrical activity and electrical activity from a ventricular ectopic beat simultaneously stimulate the ventricles. Fusion beats are indicated by a normal P-R interval and a compromised QRS complex with an appearance that is between normal and that of a QRS complex indicating ventricular tachycardia.

Atrioventricular dissociation is a form of ventricular tachycardia. It is evidenced by P waves and QRS complexes that occur at about the same rate but are unrelated. The P wave may be seen before, within, or after the QRS complex, which is usually normal in configuration. Atrioventricular dissociation is a descriptive term and not a diagnosis. The primary cause of this abnormality in impulse formation and conduction is usually digitalis toxicity.

Ventricular tachycardia and PVC are usually treated with quinidine or procainamide. But, these agents are not used when ventricular arrhythmias are secondary to congestive heart failure. In such cases, therapy includes cage rest and administration of digitalis, diuretics, morphine, and oxygen.

Animals affected with ventricular arrhythmias and presented in a comatose condition are given 2% lidocaine without epinephrine intravenously. The dosage is 2 to 4 mg/kg over one to two minutes followed by 0.5 to 2 mg/kg every 20 to 60 minutes.[1] Quinidine sulfate (6 to 20 mg/kg orally every six to eight hours) takes effect in about an hour. Procainamide is commonly used to treat ventricular arrhythmias, DC cardioversion can be used in refractive cases, but often, the arrhythmia returns.

Congestive heart failure

Congestive heart failure can either cause or be caused by ventricular tachycardia, but it usually initiates ventricular tachycardia. Patients with severe congestive heart failure usually have excessive pulmonary edema, requiring immediate treatment.

If pulmonary edema is present and the animal dyspneic, therapy includes Lasix® (Hoechst), aminophylline, and ouabain (Lilly). Hydrazaline and other hypotensive agents are used to reduce the cardiovascular load. Morphine may be given subcutaneously to quiet a dyspneic animal. Oxygen is a necessity. If the arrhythmia worsens after a digitalis derivative is administered, lidocaine should be injected in an intravenous bolus of 2 to 4 mg/kg over one to two minutes. Also, 0.5 to 2 mg/kg of lidocaine can be injected slowly every 20 to 60 minutes. The heart rate and rhythm should be monitored. In cases of ventricular-induced congestive heart failure, quinidine may be used for six to eight weeks. If possible, it should then be withdrawn gradually over a two-week period.

Ventricular fibrillation

Ventricular fibrillation is an ominous sign. Affected animals collapse without a heart beat or femoral pulse and have dilated pupils and possibly, seizures. The electrocardiogram (ECG) shows baseline undulations without specific P waves or QRS complexes.

Cardiac arrest occurs as a result of ventricular fibrillation and cardiac standstill. These abnormalities can only be differentiated with an ECG. Cardiac standstill is evidenced on the ECG by a straight baseline. The undulations of ventricular fibrillation are coarse or fine; coarse undulations indicate greater receptivity to defibrillation therapy.

Treatment of ventricular fibrillation consists of intermittent positive pressure oxygenation, internal or external cardiac massage, administration of lactated Ringer solution with sodium bicarbonate, and one to two sharp blows to the chest. If these measures elicit no response, DC cardioversion is initiated. Electric current is applied as each R wave is seen. The initial electrical charge is 2 watt-sec/kg.[1] If there is still no response, the charge is doubled.

If DC cardioversion does not convert the fibrillation, manual cardiac massage and intracardial administration of sodium bicarbonate and epinephrine are repeated. Epinephrine converts fine fibrillation to coarse, and the sodium bicarbonate reduces myocardial irritation. This treatment and DC cardioversion are alternated until some result is noted. But, if the cardiac rhythm does not improve within 10 minutes, therapy is stopped.

REFERENCE

1. Tilley, L.P.: *Essentials of Canine and Feline Electrocardiography.* C.V. Mosby Co., St. Louis, Mo., 1975.

CHAPTER 30

Treatment/ management of cardiovascular disorders

THE METHODOLOGY for conducting and interpreting electrocardiograms (ECG) has been described.[1-3] The process has been simplified further by the development of an electrocardiographic telephone service (Cardiopet, Inc., 6183 Strickland Ave., Brooklyn, N.Y.). For a minimal investment, any veterinary office equipped with a telephone may have ECGs recorded and interpreted by a veterinary cardiologist. Because treatment and management of cardiac disorders require proper and repeated use of electrocardiography, access to an in-house ECG machine or an electrocardiographic service is becoming a necessity instead of a luxury.

Congestive heart failure is defined as the inability of the heart to accept the venous return and meet the body's circulatory needs. The congestion is caused by inadequate pumping action of the heart. If the failure is in the left side of the heart, congestion occurs in the lungs, resulting in increased pulmonary venous pressure, edema, and inadequate arterial perfusion of vital organs. When there is failure in the right side of the heart, the liver, spleen, and abdominal cavity become congested. Hepatomegaly, splenomegaly, and ascites result. Because the right side of the heart is unable to adequately pump blood through the pulmonary circulation, the vital organs become hypoxic. If there is insufficient perfusion in cases of left heart failure or peripheral venous congestion in cases of right heart failure, sodium and water are retained. Heart failure in dogs most commonly occurs secondary to chronic mitral valvular fibrosis. This disease process can be classified into four phases:

Phase I: No clinical signs are noted, and the animal is in cardiac compensation.

Phase II: Clinical signs are seen only after moderate exercise. Coughing may occur at night. Only the left side of the heart is involved.

Phase III: After mild exercise, there are clinical signs and paroxysmal pulmonary edema. Involvement of the left side of the heart is more pronounced.

Phase IV: Clinical signs and near constant pulmonary edema occur even during rest periods. Eventually, right heart failure with ascites and edema result.

Treatment of acute congestive heart failure

The primary objectives in treating acute phase IV congestive heart failure are to 1) relieve anxiety, 2) relieve respiratory distress and improve oxygenation of the blood, 3) increase the heart's pumping ability, thereby improving perfusion to vital organs, and 4) treat the cause of the condition.

Patients with acute congestive heart failure are usually distressed, apprehensive, and dyspneic. They should be placed in an oxygen cage or given oxygen via mask. Further treatment should include:

1. Morphine at a dose of 1.0 to 2.0 mg/kg subcutaneously to relieve anxiety and decrease oxygen requirements.

2. Furosemide (Lasix® —Hoechst-Roussel) at a dosage of 2 to 4 mg/kg, intravenously or subcutaneously, every 4 to 12 hours as needed to relieve pulmonary edema.

3. Bronchodilators such as aminophylline (Aminophyllin® —Searle) or theophylline (Theophyl® —Knoll) given at a dosage of 6 to 10 mg/kg intravenously or intramuscularly every six to eight hours as needed. (For intravenous use these drugs should be diluted in 20 ml normal saline solution and given slowly. They are potent vasodilators and, thus, must be administered with caution if given intravenously, especially in cats.)

4. Sodium bicarbonate can be given intravenously at a rate of 2 mEq/kg over a four- to eight-hour period to correct acidosis. To prevent sodium overload and paradoxal central nervous system acidosis, avoid rapid alkalization.

5. After initial stabilization, record an ECG and begin oral cardiac glycoside treatment.

Intravenous digitalization should only be done during constant ECG monitoring and by an experienced clinician. A suggested rapid oral digitalization regimen is 0.02 to 0.06 mg/kg of digoxin divided into two doses given 12 hours apart.[4] After this, maintenance levels of digoxin should be given. The dosage should be adjusted as indicated by clinical response and the ECG. A prolonged P-R interval is the normal response to cardiac glycoside therapy.

TABLE 1—ABCDs of Cardiac Resuscitation

A. Airway: Establish and maintain a patent airway by endotracheal intubation.

B. Breath: Begin intermittent, positive-pressure breathing for the animal at a rate of one breath/5 seconds.

C. Circulation: Begin external cardiac compression at a rate of 60 compressions/minute. The animal should be ventilated once every 12th compression.

D. Drugs:
1. Epinephrine intracardially at a dose of 0.1 to 0.5 mg/15 kg.
2. Sodium bicarbonate intracardially or intravenously at a rate of 1 to 2 mEq/kg, if the heart begins beating.
3. Calcium: 1.5 to 2.0 ml of 10% calcium chloride/15 kg or 6 to 8 ml of 10% calcium gluconate/15 kg.
4. Lactated Ringer solution: 40 ml/kg in dogs and 20 ml/kg in cats.

Signs of glycoside toxicity include second- or third-degree atrioventricular blocks, ventricular ectopic beats, and/or atrial tachycardia. Clinical signs of toxicity are nausea, vomiting, and diarrhea. Digoxin is excreted renally, and digitoxin is excreted hepatically. Thus, the functional ability of these organs may influence the choice of cardiac glycoside. In cases of renal failure, digitoxin should be used. If hepatic failure exists, digoxin is the treatment of choice.

Vasodilator therapy has recently received attention as adjunctive therapy in cases of congestive heart failure. Venous vasodilators increase vascular capacitance and decrease venous pressure and formation of edema. Arterial vasodilators counteract reflex vasoconstriction, decrease impedance to arterial flow, and improve tissue perfusion. The primary adverse side effect of vasodilator therapy is hypotension. Thus, dosage of these drugs should be low initially and then gradually increased to effect.

Common vasodilators are topical 2% nitroglycerine ointment (0.25 to 0.5 inch two to three times daily, use gloves to apply), hydralazine (0.5 to 2 mg/kg orally two to three times daily), and prazosin (1 to 2 mg/kg orally two to three times daily).

Additional therapy for patients with congestive heart failure includes restriction of the amount of sodium in the diet. Commercial or homemade diets may be used. Prescription Diet h/d (Hills) is adequately sodium restricted but does not seem to be palatable. Homemade diets should contain no more than 6 mg of sodium/lb of body weight/day.

Bradyarrhythmias

Bradyarrhythmias are associated with heart rates of less than 70 beats/min. and include sinus (atrial) bradycardia, sinus arrest, junctional and ventricular escape rhythms, and heart blocks. Treatment of bradycardia depends on its type and cause.

In the case of bradycardias secondary to systemic diseases causing hyperkalemia (*e.g.* renal failure and Addison disease), the specific disease process must be treated. Vagal stimulation and drug-induced bradycardias are usually responsive to atropine given at a dosage of 0.02 mg/kg three times daily, subcutaneously or orally. Isoproterenol (Isuprel® —Winthrop) is a temporary treatment for second- and third-degree heart block bradycardia. One milligram of isoproterenol in 200 ml of 5% dextrose is given in a slow drip to effect. Permanent correction of serious conduction disorders may require implantation of a pacemaker.

Tachyarrhythmias

Tachyarrhythmias are associated with a heart rate greater than 160 beats/min. and include atrial flutter, atrial tachycardia, atrial fibrillation, junctional and ventricular tachycardia, and premature ventricular contractions. Digoxin is the drug of choice for treating tachyarrhythmias arising from the atrium. Slow, oral digitalization with digoxin at maintenance dosage is the safest treatment, and clinical digitalization occurs in about 7 to 10 days. If digoxin fails to halt the arrhythmia, then propranolol (Inderal® Ayerst) can be given by mouth at a dosage of 10 to 40 mg three times daily. Because propranolol can be hepatotoxic, caution should be used in cases requiring long-term therapy.

In severe cases of tachyarrhythmia such as premature ventricular contraction and ventricular tachycardia, digoxin should be withdrawn and lidocaine used as a short-acting myocardial depressant. The recommended dosage of lidocaine is 2 mg/kg intravenously over two to four minutes or 25 to 40 mg per 30-minute period in a dextrose drip. Lidocaine with epinephrine should not be used. For long-term myocardial depression, procainamide (Pronestyl® —Squibb) is preferred at a dosage of 6 to 20 mg/kg by mouth every 8 to 12 hours. Quinidine (Quinidine® —Lilly) is often used, but results are unpredictable. The common dosage is 6 to 20 mg/kg orally every six to eight hours. Phenytoin sodium (Dilantin® —Parke Davis) is safe and effective for treating tachyarrhythmias and digitalis-induced arrhythmia. The common dosage is 50 to 150 mg intravenously, not to exceed 50 mg/min. for short-term, serious arrhythmias.

Cardiopulmonary resuscitation

Cardiopulmonary resuscitation is necessary whenever cardiac arrest occurs. Cardiac arrest is defined as an absence of cardiac output, and successful resuscitation requires early (within three to five minutes), vigorous and effective therapy. The American Animal Hospital Association (AAHA) publishes a Cardiac Emergency Chart listing the proper steps to take in cases of cardiac arrest. Every small animal practitioner should keep this chart near an emergency kit containing drugs recommended by the AAHA cardiology committee. Table 1 briefly outlines the process of cardiac resuscitation.

REFERENCES

1. Wilkes, R.D. *et al*: Electrocardiography-1: A Systemic Approach to Obtaining an Electrocardiograph. *VM/SAC* 77(3):342-346; 1982.
2. Wilkes, R.D. *et al*: Electrocardiography-2: Supraventricular Arrhythmias. *VM/SAC* 77(4):510-513; 1982.
3. Wilkes, R.D. *et al*: Electrocardiography-3: Ventricular Arrhythmias. *VM/SAC* 77(5):690-691; 1982.
4. Bonagura, J.: Acute Heart Failure. In *Current Veterinary Therapy VII* (R.W. Kirk, Ed.). W.B. Saunders, Philadelphia, Pa., 1980; pp 359-367.

8 Immunology for the practitioner

CHAPTER 31

Normal/abnormal immune responses & systemic immune-mediated diseases

THE NORMAL IMMUNE RESPONSE of animals is protective and beneficial. It is designed to prevent disease after exposure to infectious and parasitic organisms, cancer cells, and other foreign antigenic substances. However, the immune response becomes abnormal and deleterious when it causes autoimmunity, immunodeficiency, and allergic disorders. These abnormal immune responses can lead to systemic immune-mediated disorders such as autoimmune hemolytic anemia, immune-mediated thrombocytopenia, and systemic lupus erythematosus. Results of routine laboratory tests may lead one to suspect these diseases. However, specific immunologic tests (*e.g.* direct Coombs test, platelet factor 3 [PF-3] test, antinuclear antibody [ANA] test, and the lupus erythematosus [LE] cell test) are needed to confirm the diagnosis.

Normal immune response

In the normal immune response, the animal reacts to exposure to foreign antigens (*e.g.* viruses, bacteria, parasites, fungi, cancer cells) by producing specific antibodies and/or cytotoxic cells to remore or neutralize the antigens. An *antigen* is a substance that induces an immune reaction by a cellular and/or a humoral component of the immune system. Future encounters with that specific antigen result in an augmented or anamnestic immune response.

In dogs, all antigenic substances present on the 42nd day *in utero* are recognized as "self," and any antigenic substances the body is exposed to after that time are considered foreign. Normally, an immune response is mounted against any foreign antigens. The loss of the ability to distinguish between the body's own tissues and foreign antigens results in the development of autoimmune diseases. Loss of the ability to establish or maintain a normal immune response leads to immunodeficiency diseases. The hereditary predisposition to form reaginic antibody (IgE) is a cause of allergic diseases.

Antibodies are globulin protein produced by the humoral component of the immune system in response to antigenic stimulation. More specifically, these antibodies are called *immunoglobulins.* In companion animals, there are four major classes of immunoglobulins: IgG, IgA, IgM, and IgE.

The principal immunoglobulin produced by the immune system is IgG; about 80% of all antibacterial, antiviral, and antitoxin immunoglobulins belong to this class. IgA, the primary secretory immunoglobulin, is active at mucosal surfaces, *e.g.* along the respiratory tract, gastrointestinal tract, and urogenital system. IgM is the initial immunoglobulin produced after antigenic stimulation and is most important in early protection against disease. In animals genetically susceptible to allergic disorders, excessive amounts of IgE, or reaginic immunoglobulin, are produced after exposure to substances that are innocuous to most individuals.

The complement system, which helps the immune system destroy foreign antigens, comprises 12 serum proteins. These proteins react in an integrated sequence after being activated by IgG or IgM. The result is lysis of the membrane of the target bacterial cell.

The immune system consists of three primary groups of cells: T-lymphocytes, B-lymphocytes, and macrophages. The T-lymphocytes, which are derived from the thymus, cannot produce antibody but can proliferate in response to an antigen. When stimulated by an antigen, they become regulatory, effector, or recognition (memory) T-lymphocytes. Regulatory T-lymphocytes become either helper T-cells, expediting the antibody response of B-lymphocytes, or suppressor T-cells, suppressing this response. Effector T-lymphocytes proliferate and either 1) produce chemicals, *i.e.* lymphokines, that are destructive to the antigen or 2) become killer T-cells that destroy the antigens by direct contact. This is one of the body's major immunologic protective mechanisms against cancer cells. Recognition T-lymphocytes "remember" an antigen that has previously been introduced into the body. Of the lymphocytes circulating in the blood, 80% are T-lymphocytes. These cells also circulate through the interstitial extravascular areas of the skin, kidneys, gonads, and uterus.

B-lymphocytes are derived from bone marrow. When antigenically stimulated, they either 1) transform into plasma cells and produce specific antibody against the antigen, or 2) become recognition (memory) B-lymphocytes serving the same function as recognition T-lymphocytes. Only about 20% of the lymphocytes in the blood are B-lymphocytes. After their transformation into plasma cells, they usually remain in the sinuses of the secondary lymphoid tissues, *i.e.* spleen and lymph nodes, and secrete antibody into the lymph fluid.

The third type of cell required to effect an immune response is an accessory or adherent cell. These cells are nonlymphoid, macrophage-like cells derived from bone marrow. They process the antigen and present it to the lymphocytes, thus initiating antibody production by B-lymphocytes and/or lymphokine production by T-lymphocytes.

Abnormal immune responses

Four reactions have been described whereby the immune system damages the body's own tissues and causes disease. They are designated Types I through IV.

Type I (anaphylaxis) reactions

These reactions are caused by the release of pharmacologically active substances (*e.g.* histamine, serotonin, and bradykinins) from mast cells and/or basophils. The release of these substances is triggered by antigens binding to specific antibodies (IgE) on the mast cell/basophil membranes. Many types of antigens including insect venoms, pollens, and antibiotics, can cause such a reaction.

The anaphylactic reaction is immediate and may affect the 1) respiratory system, causing pulmonary edema, laryngeal edema, and bronchospasms; 2) gastrointestinal system, resulting in vomiting and/or diarrhea; or 3) skin, causing urticaria. Common disease processes seen with this type of reaction are allergic inhalant dermatitis (atopy), allergic rhinitis, allergic bronchitis, and allergic enteritis (food allergy). A hereditary predisposition exists for producing high levels of IgE; thus allergic diseases are heritable.

Type II reactions

Reactions of this type probably are the most common abnormal immune responses. In this type of reaction, specific antibodies and complement bind with antigens that are attached to the surface of the host's normal cells, causing immune destruction of these cells. Some diseases associated with this reaction are autoimmune hemolytic anemia, immune-mediated thrombocytopenia, the pemphigus skin diseases (*e.g. Pemphigus vulgaris, P. foliaceus, P. vegetans, P. erythematosus*, and bullous pemphigoid), and myasthenia gravis.

Type III reactions

These occur when copious amounts of antigen, antibody, and complement are deposited in the walls of blood vessels in highly vascular tissues. These deposits physically impair function and attract phagocytes, which further damage the host's tissues by releasing lysosomal enzymes. Disease syndromes resulting from this type of injury are immune-complex glomerulonephritis associated with systemic lupus erythematosus, rheumatoid arthritis, and immune-mediated uveitis.

Type IV reactions

These reactions are the result of cell-mediated immunity whereby sensitized T-lymphocytes react directly with the sensitizing antigen. After this reaction, the lymphocytes release lymphokines that attempt to destroy the sensitizing antigen, thus activating macrophages and an inflammatory response. The antigens that most commonly stimulate this type of reaction are the systemic fungal organisms, mycobacteria, and feline corona virus. Inflammatory immune-mediated granulomas are a sequela of the injury.

TABLE 1—Procedures for Performing the Direct Coombs Test

1. Collect a blood sample in a tube containing heparin or EDTA.
2. Separate out the erythrocytes and wash them twice in isotonic phosphate-buffered saline solution.
3. In small tubes, make serial twofold dilutions of 0.2 ml of species-specific anti-IgG, anti-IgM, and anti-C_3 until they reach a 1:32 dilution.
4. Add to the tubes 0.2 ml of a 2% suspension of the washed erythrocytes. Gently shake the tubes and incubate at 37 C for 60 minutes.
5. Make another set of the same dilutions given in steps 3 and 4 and incubate the tubes at 4 C for 60 minutes to check for cold-agglutinins.
6. Observe the cells macroscopically for agglutination.
7. Using a scale of 0 (negative) to +4, grade the results, based on the strength of the agglutination.

Systemic immune-mediated diseases

Autoimmune hemolytic anemia (AIHA)

This disease results when the immune system destroys the body's erythrocytes. The disease process, which may be acute or chronic with a sudden or insidious onset, affects both dogs and cats. No age or breed of animal seems predisposed to the disease, but it is more common in females than males. Clinical signs are those usually associated with anemia and intravascular hemolysis including weakness, pale mucous membranes, icterus, and splenomegaly. Clinicopathologic findings are a Coombs-positive, regenerative anemia with spherocytosis. Laboratory diagnosis and classifications of anemias have been described.[1-4]

The direct Coombs test is definitive for diagnosing AIHA. This test uses species-specific antibodies against IgG, IgM, and C_3 (the third component of complement) to detect autoantibodies attached to the membranes of the erythrocytes.

The procedures for performing the direct Coombs test are listed in Table 1. The test is reliable, but false positives can occur in cases of lymphoreticular neoplasias and after blood transfusions. False negatives may result if the AIHA is in remission and after therapy with corticosteroids or other immunosuppressive drugs. In addition to the direct Coombs test, the indirect Coombs test is used to detect anti-erythrocyte antibody in man. The latter test is not valid for use in veterinary medicine.

Immune-mediated thrombocytopenia

Formerly known as idiopathic thrombocytopenia purpura, this disease is caused by immunologic destruction of the body's blood platelets. Both dogs and cats can be affected by the disease, though in cats it is most often associated with infection by feline leukemia virus. The disease is seen more frequently in females than males. However, no predisposition by age or breed has been noted. Common clinical signs are petechial and ecchymotic hemorrhages, epistaxis, and eventually, anemia. The condition may occur acutely, chronically or cyclically, but hemorrhage usually develops spontaneously when the platelet count falls below 50,000/cubic millimeter. Laboratory techniques for evaluating platelet function and counting platelets have been described.[5]

The best way to confirm immune-mediated thrombocytopenia is to demonstrate anti-platelet antibody by means of the platelet factor 3 (PF-3) test.[6] In this test, platelets from a healthy dog are mixed with canine-contact product (activated clotting factor XI and XII) and placed in two tubes. One of these tubes contains 0.1 ml of the patient's serum; the other contains 0.1 ml of serum from a clinically normal dog. The tubes are incubated at 37 C for five minutes, then 0.025 M calcium chloride is added to each tube. If anti-platelet antibody is in the patient's serum, the clotting time is shortened by at least 10 seconds, as compared to the normal serum. False negatives can occur if the patient has been given corticosteroids or other immunosuppressive drugs.

Many cases of immune-mediated thrombocytopenia fail to show positive results for a PF-3 test. In such cases, when the disease is still suspected or when the PF-3 test cannot be done, samples of bone marrow should be examined. If megakaryocytes, the precursor cells to platelets, are detected and ehrlichiosis can be ruled out, the patient should be given glucocorticoids. A presumptive diagnosis of immune-mediated thrombocytopenia can be based on a good response to therapy. Techniques for examining bone marrow and demonstrating megakaryocytes have been described.[7]

Systemic lupus erythematosus (SLE)

This is a multi-systemic inflammatory disease that can involve the skin, kidneys, musculoskeletal system, and blood. The onset may be acute, chronic, or cyclic. Clinical signs depend on the organs affected, but the most common sign is malaise accompanied by a fever that does not respond to antibiotic therapy. When the skin is involved, the most characteristic lesions are profound erythema and crusting and alopecia of the nasal area, feet, and ears. A more generalized distribution of lesions, with the lesions varying from seborrhea to ulcers, has been reported in recent cases involving both dogs and cats. If the blood is involved, AIHA and/or immune-mediated thrombocytopenia may occur concomitantly with SLE.

When SLE affects the musculoskeletal system, polymyositis and/or polyarthritis may be characterized by lameness shifting from one leg to another, stilted gait, signs of pain, and progressive

TABLE 2—Procedures for Performing the Antinuclear Antibody Test

1. First perform the test using a dilution of 1:10 on the patient's serum and a known positive and a known negative control.
2. Place the patient's diluted serum and the controls on separate slides, each containing nonspecies-specific cell substrate. Incubate the slides at room temperature for 15 minutes.
3. Wash the slides with two changes of phosphate-buffered saline solution for 30 minutes. Next, overlay the slides with fluorescein-conjugated, species-specific anti-IgG and allow them to incubate for 15 minutes.
4. Wash the slides in three changes of phosphate-buffered saline solution for 45 minutes and rinse them in distilled water.
5. Examine the slides under a fluorescent microscope.
6. If the 1:10 dilution is positive, the test should be titered out by serial dilutions until the highest positive dilution (titer) is obtained.

muscle wasting. Radiographs of long bones frequently reveal a nonerosive polyarthritis. Culture and cytology of joint fluid usually reveal a sterile fluid in which small lymphocytes predominate. Exfoliative cytologic techniques for evaluating joint and other body fluids have been described.[8] When the kidneys are involved, SLE usually is manifested as a protein-losing glomerulonephritis caused by excess deposits of antigen-antibody-complement complex in the vascular walls of the glomeruli.

Systemic lupus erythematosus is an immune-mediated disease in which antibodies are formed against the nucleoproteins and other nuclear and cytoplasmic antigens of the host's cells. Because antinuclear antibodies are usually detectable, the ANA test is a major diagnostic test for systemic lupus erythematosus. The antinuclear antibodies are not species-specific; therefore any cell substrate with many nuclei can be used, *e.g.* mouse liver cells, tissue-cultured human epithelial cells, and recently a protozoon (*Crithidia lucidae*) that has a kinetoplast composed of pure double-stranded deoxyribonucleic acid. The procedure for performing the ANA test is given in Table 2. Titers compatible with a diagnosis of SLE vary somewhat, depending on the laboratory procedure used. Generally, however, titers greater than 1:100 are considered positive, titers between 1:50 and 1:100 are questionable, and titers less than 1:50 are considered negative.

Another widely used immunologic test for diagnosing SLE is the LE cell test. Lupus erythematosus cells are phagocytes that have phagocytized an ANA-coated homogenous mass of nuclear material from degenerating leukocytes. The LE cell test requires 5 ml of fresh clotted blood. This blood is allowed to incubate for two hours at 37 C and then is strained through a wire mesh. After incubating at 37 C for 30 more minutes, the blood is centrifuged. Smears made from the buffy coat are stained with Wright stain and examined for LE cells. A finding of four LE cells per slide is considered positive, and eight cells is strongly positive. The LE cell test is much less accurate than the ANA test. False negatives often occur when even small amounts of glucocorticoids have been administered exogenously.

Because they are complex and require special reagents, the direct Coombs, PF-3, and ANA tests are usually done by reference or commercial laboratories. Reagents for these tests can be obtained from Miles Scientific Laboratories, 30W475 North Aurora Road, Naperville, Illinois 60566.

REFERENCES

1. Goldston, R.T. *et al*: The Clinical Pathology Laboratory - 3; Evaluation of the Erythrocytes: Hematocrit and Hemaglobin Determinations. *VM/SAC* 75(3):407-410; 1980.
2. Goldston, R.T. *et al*: The Clinical Pathology Laboratory - 4; Evaluation of the Erythrocytes: Total Erythrocyte Indices and Sedimentation Rate. *VM/SAC* 75(4):586-590; 1980.
3. Seybold, I.M. *et al*: The Clinical Pathology Laboratory - 5; Evaluation of the Blood Smear. *VM/SAC* 75(5):781-790; 1980.
4. Goldston, R.T. *et al*: The Clinical Pathology Laboratory - 6; Anemias. *VM/SAC* 75(6):973-977; 1980.
5. Goldston, R.T. *et al*: The Clinical Pathology Laboratory - 32; Hemostasis/Coagulation: A Clinical Approach to Bleeding Disorders. *VM/SAC* 77(8): 1982.
6. Wilkins, R.J. *et al*: Immunologically Mediated Thrombocytopenia in the Dog. *JAVMA* *163*:277; 1973.
7. Seybold, I.M. *et al*: The Clinical Pathology Laboratory - 10; Examination of the Bone Marrow. *VM/SAC* 75(10):1517-1521; 1980.
8. Seybold, I.M. *et al*: The Clinical Pathology Laboratory - 31; Exfoliative Cytology. *VM/SAC* 77(7):1029-1033; 1982.

CHAPTER 32

Intradermal skin testing for allergic inhalant dermatitis

ALLERGIC INHALANT DERMATITIS (AID) is a chronic, progressive heritable dermatosis resulting from hypersensitivity to inhaled allergens (antigens). The principal sign of the disease is pruritus involving primarily the feet, face, ears, and axillae. Affected dogs typically lick, rub, or scratch these areas. In general, clinical signs become evident when an animal is 1 to 3 years of age. Initially, the animal is symptomatic only seasonally, when the offending pollens are present in highest concentrations. However, signs may persist throughout the year in some cases, particularly when the allergens are house dust, molds, wool, or kapok.

The disease affects 10% of all dogs. It is seen most frequently in Dalmatians, Irish Setters, and terriers, particularly West Highland Terriers and Cairn Terriers. The incidence of AID is higher in females than in males.

Diagnosis of AID is made on the basis of the history and clinical signs and by ruling out other pruritic dermatoses. The diagnosis can usually be confirmed by intradermal skin testing.

Food allergy dermatitis can be determined by feeding the animal a hypoallergenic diet consisting only of mutton and rice (Prescription Diet® d/d® — Hill's) for at least a month. A significant reduction in the pruritus indicates that food allergy is contributing to the dermatitis. Food allergy dermatitis is especially likely if clinical signs are accompanied by minor gastrointestinal disturbances such as flatulence and/or periodic diarrhea. However, many dogs with food allergies show no gastrointestinal signs.

Other pruritic dermatoses such as flea allergy dermatitis, scabies, dermatomycosis, and pelodera dermatitis can be ruled out by physical examination and microscopic examination of skin scrapings, fungal and bacterial cultures, and biopsy specimens of skin.

Intradermal skin test

The intradermal skin test is the most reliable, readily available method for diagnosing AID and identifying specific allergens. The best time to perform the test is when the patient is most symptomatic and has not been given oral corticosteroids for two to three weeks or long-acting injectable corticosteroids for five to six weeks. The dog should not receive antihistamines, tranquilizers, or progesterone for five to seven days before testing.

The allergens (antigens)

The specific allergens selected for intradermal testing and subsequent hyposensitization vary, depending on the practitioner's geographic location and on the patient's particular environment. Local and state agriculture departments and county agriculture agents can advise practitioners concerning common pollens in the area and seasons of highest pollen concentration. Commercial suppliers of antigens also provide such information on a regional basis. Finally, consultation with a local allergist may yield useful information on the selection of appropriate antigens. Antigens used in our practice are listed in Table 1. Group mixtures of antigens can be used to test for sensitivity to molds and grass pollens because they cross-react well. Tree pollens and weed pollens should not be used in group mixtures because they cross-react poorly.

Antigens for testing and hyposensitization can be purchased from any of several commercial laboratories such as Greer Laboratories (Lenoir, N.C.), Center Laboratories (Port Washington, N.Y.), Hollister-Stier Laboratories (Atlanta, Ga.), and Dome Laboratories (West Haven, Conn.). The antigens are available in several forms (*e.g.* aqueous extract, alum-precipitated extract) and concentrations (*e.g.* 10,000, 20,000, and 40,000 protein nitrogen units (PNU)/ml). We recommend the aqueous extract in a stock dilution of 20,000 PNU/milliliter. This concentration has a shelf life of one to two years and is easy to dilute for testing and hyposensitization. Stock antigens should be numbered and refrigerated. Extreme care should be taken to prevent cross-contamination of antigens.

For intradermal testing, stock antigens are diluted to a concentration of 1,000 PNU/milliliter. At this concentration, the antigen has a shelf life of only one month. Therefore, only small quantities should be diluted at one time. Antigens that are not measured in PNUs are diluted to 1:1000 weight/volume (w/v). The diluent is phosphate-buffered saline solution. It can be purchased in small sterile vials from companies that supply antigens.

TABLE 1—Antigens Used at Animal Hospital of St. Petersburg, Fla.

Histamine Sulfate (positive control)
Saline Solution (negative control)
House Dust
House Dust, Mattress, Rug, Upholstery (HMRU)
Kapok
Sheep Wool
Feather Mix
Flea
Mold Mix No. 1
Alternaria tenus, Hormodendrum hordei, Helminthosporium sativum, Aspergillus niger, Penicillium notatum
Mold Mix No. 2
Curvularia spicifera, Fusarium moniliforme, Pullularia pullulans, Mucor plumbeus, Rhizopus nigricans

Slash Pine	Bermuda-Johnson Mix
Coconut/Queen Palm	Bahia
Live Oak	Salt Grass
American Elm	Yellow Dock—Sorrel Mix
Hickory Mix	Lambs Quarter
Eastern Sycamore	Dog Fennel
Sweet Gum	English Plantain
Mango	Pigweed
Red Mulberry	Ragweed Mix
Melaleuca Pollen	Baccharis
Orange Pollen	Bald Cypress
Pepper Tree	Bayberry (myrtle)
Beefwood/Australian Pine	Marsh Elder

The test procedure

Intradermal testing is done with the patient in lateral recumbency. Chemical restraint, *i.e.* tranquilizers or anesthetics, should be avoided because they can alter the patient's reactions. If the dog is difficult to handle, have the owner present during testing to calm it.

An area of the lateral chest and abdomen is gently clipped with a No. 40 clipper blade, care being taken not to cause erythema or inflammation of the skin. The clipped area should not be washed or scrubbed. Each injection site is numbered with an indelible marking pen, and each vial of antigen is marked with the corresponding number.

A tuberculin syringe with a 26-gauge, 3/8-in. needle and an intradermal bevel is used to inject 0.1 ml (*i.e.* 100 PNU) of test antigen, which has been diluted to 1,000 PNU/ml or 1:1,000 w/v. The injections are given intradermally at as uniform a depth as possible. Antigens that are also irritants, *e.g.* house dust, kapok, household insects, and fleas are diluted to 250 PNU/ml and the patient is given a 0.1-ml (25-PNU) injection of the antigen. This is done to ensure that any skin reaction is due to allergic hypersensitivity and not physical irritation.

A negative control (0.1 ml of phosphate-buffered saline solution) is injected as is a positive control (0.1 ml of a 1:100,000 dilution of histamine

TABLE 2—Schedule for Hyposensitization

Day Number	Vial No. 1 (100-200 PNU/ml)	Vial No. 2 (1,000-2,000 PNU/ml)	Vial No. 3 (10,000-20,000 PNU/ml)
0	0.1 ml		
3	0.2 ml		
6	0.4 ml		
9	0.8 ml		
12		0.1 ml	
15		0.2 ml	
18		0.4 ml	
21		0.8 ml	
24			0.1 ml
27			0.2 ml
30			0.4 ml
33			0.8 ml
36			1.0 ml
46			1.0 ml
66	Continue with 1.0 ml Vial No. 3 every 14 days		

phosphate [Center Laboratorics]). Reactions are read at 5, 10, 15, and 30 minutes. Each site where antigen was injected is compared with the positive and negative control sites. Formation of a wheal about one-third the size of the wheal produced by the positive control is considered a positive reaction. These reactions are measured on a scale of +1 to +4, with +4 being the size of the wheal caused by injection of the histamine phosphate.

False positive reactions can occur if the antigen is contaminated with bacteria or is insufficiently diluted. Irritants in the antigen or diluent may also produce false positive reactions. False negative reactions can result if the antigen is injected subcutaneously or with air or when the antigen is outdated or overly diluted. False negatives may also be caused by 1) exogenous interference such as that resulting from administration of corticosteroids, antihistamines, progestins, or tranquilizers; or 2) endogenous interference, *e.g.* hyperanxiety causing release of epinephrine, pregnancy resulting in increased amounts of progestin, or Cushing disease causing elevated levels of glucocorticoids.

Once the patient's sensitivities are known, as many of the offending allergens as possible should be removed from the patient's environment. Frequently, this is impossible except when the allergen is wool, feathers, or some other household item. Fleas can also be eliminated from the household environment. Some clients, when shown their pet's reaction to fleas, step up programs to control the pests.

Hyposensitization

If an allergen 1) cannot be removed from the environment and 2) produced a +3 or +4 intradermal reaction, it should be used for hyposensitization. However, the number of allergens used should be limited to 10 or fewer. This reduces the possibility of an overload reaction and prevents dilution of antigens to the point of immunologic inactivity. If the dog reacts to more than 10 allergens, selection depends on the animal's history and environment.

Hyposensitization is based on the theory that when allergens are injected into the body, they form blocking IgG antibodies. These antibodies can bind inhaled allergens before they react with the IgE antibodies on the surface of the mast cells in the skin and cause an allergic reaction.

Other important theories of allergic disease are the *threshold phenomenon* and the *summation of effect* concept. The first theory states that an individual can tolerate a certain load of allergens without manifesting any allergic disease. However, a small increase in that load may push the individual over the *threshold*, causing clinical signs. According to the summation of effect theory, concomitant pruritic disorders may also push an animal over its pruritic threshold. Therefore, all factors contributing to the pruritus such as flea allergy, food allergy, and pyoderma must be treated while the patient is being hyposensitized.

The antigen mixture for hyposensitization is prepared in three vials. Sterile, empty vials can be obtained from suppliers of antigens. Vial No. 3, the maintenance vial, is filled with 20 ml of antigen mixture that has been diluted to a concentration of 10,000 to 20,000 PNU/milliliter. Thus, if the patient requires 10 allergens, 2 ml of the stock solution (20,000 PNU/ml) of each of the chosen allergens is added to the vial. This provides 20 ml of solution containing 20,000 PNU of antigen/milliliter. If the patient requires five antigens, then 2 ml of the stock solution of each is added to the vial with 10 ml of phosphate-buffered saline solution. This provides 20 ml of solution containing 10,000 PNU of antigen/milliliter.

Vial No. 2 is made by adding 0.5 ml of the solution in Vial No. 3 to 4.5 ml of phosphate-buffered saline solution. Vial No. 1 is prepared by adding 0.5 ml of the mixture in Vial No. 2 to 4.5 ml of phosphate-buffered saline solution.

The hyposensitization program is started by giving small doses of Vial No. 1 and gradually increasing the volume of the injection to 1.0 milliliter. This process is repeated for Vial Nos. 2 and 3 until the patient is receiving a maximum dose of 1.0 ml of the solution in Vial No. 3 every two weeks. The hyposensitization schedule is outlined in Table 2. The injections may be given subcutaneously at home by the client, who should be given complete instructions.

A successful hyposensitization program depends on an accurate diagnosis, proper identification of offending allergens, a conscientious owner, good communications with the client, and a controllable animal. The client should be informed that successful hyposensitization may require one to two years of treatment and that the procedure is not always effective. Generally, one-third of cases respond very well, requiring little or no further corticosteroid therapy, one-third have a variable response and require periodic corticosteroid therapy at a reduced dosage and frequency, and one-third show little or no response. Intradermal skin testing and hyposensitization has proved ineffective for patients with food allergies.

Comment

Intradermal skin testing and hyposensitization are in-hospital procedures that can be performed in even the most basic laboratory.

CHAPTER 33

Practical bacteriology

Bacteriology is a field of veterinary medicine that has been left mainly to large diagnostic laboratories because of misconceptions about excessive cost, complexity, and time involved with an in-hospital microbiology laboratory. If the practitioner limited the in-hospital culturing to specimens taken from the eyes, ears, skin, urine, vagina, and abscesses, the cost and time involved would be kept within an acceptable level.

Veterinary technicians may also be capable of isolating and identifying the most common bacterial pathogens with a small amount of training. Specimens requiring anaerobic culture techniques and isolates that are not recognized should be sent to a diagnostic laboratory.

The reagents and equipment needed to set up in-house microbiology include:

1) Incubator
2) Sensi-Disk® (Becton-Dickinson) dispenser (twelve-disk dispenser for use with 150 mm plates)
3) Inoculating loops
4) Sterile swabs
5) Media
   a) MacConkey agar or MacConkey/blood agar
   b) Blood agar split plates
   c) Mueller-Hinton agar
   d) Thioglycolate nutrient broth (Thio)
6) Antibiotic sensitivity disks
7) ONPG (O-nitrophenyl-beta-D-galactopyranoside), citrate, and urea disks.
8) Taxo N® Disks (Becton-Dickinson) or cytochrome oxidase disks
9) 3% potassium hydroxide (KOH)
10) 3% hydrogen peroxide (H_2O_2)
11) Plasma from EDTA tubes ($<$24 hours old)
12) Thermometer (–20 to 110 C)
13) Sterile polystyrene culture plates if agar is to be made in-hospital
14) Gram staining kit
15) Bunsen burner

Initially, prepackaged agars should be used until the practitioner feels the in-hospital laboratory results will not be compromised by making agars from packages of powder.

Organisms commonly isolated from various organs and structures are listed in Tables 1-6.

After a sample is collected with a sterile swab, a Gram stain (*Figure 1*) is performed. Primary isolation of the organism is begun by swabbing one fourth of the surface of blood and MacConkey agar plates. To obtain isolated colonies, a sterile inoculating loop and the triple-streak method are used. By streaking in three different directions and never repeating an area, organisms are diluted over the entire plate. The plates are incubated in an inverted position for 24 hours at 35 to 37 centigrade.

Figure 1 — Gram staining

1) After applying smear, (a small amount of sample to a clean slide) allow it to air dry then gently fix by applying a small amount of heat.
2) Stain slide with crystal or methyl violet, 1½ – 2 min.
3) Wash with iodine-potassium solution (mordant), 1 min.
4) Wash and decolorize with acetone or alcohol, few seconds.
5) Counterstain with carbol-fuchsin or safranin, 1½ – 1 min.

Note: Wash slide with water between each step.
Gram-positive = deep violet
Gram-negative = red to pink
Doubtful stains = usually Gram-positive

If no growth is noted re-incubation for another 24 hours is necessary. If a fastidious organism such as *Corynebacterium* or *Streptococcus* is suspected, a culture tube of Thio broth should be inoculated initially and subcultured onto a plate if growth appears. If organisms were seen on the Gram stain, but no growth is obtained on the culture media, the sample should be forwarded to a diagnostic laboratory.

At 24 hours, all distinct colonies on blood and MacConkey agar plates should be examined for size, shape, smoothness, creaminess, etc. Each distinct colony should be Gram stained and tested as

TABLE 1—Bacteria Commonly Involved in Urinary Infections

Proteus spp	*Streptococcus* spp
Pseudomonas spp	*Enterobacter* spp
Staphylococcus spp	*Corynebacterium* spp
Escherichia coli spp	

TABLE 4—Microbial Agents Commonly Involved in Eye INfections

Streptococcus spp	*Chlamydia* spp
Staphylococcus spp	Certain viral agents

Figure 2

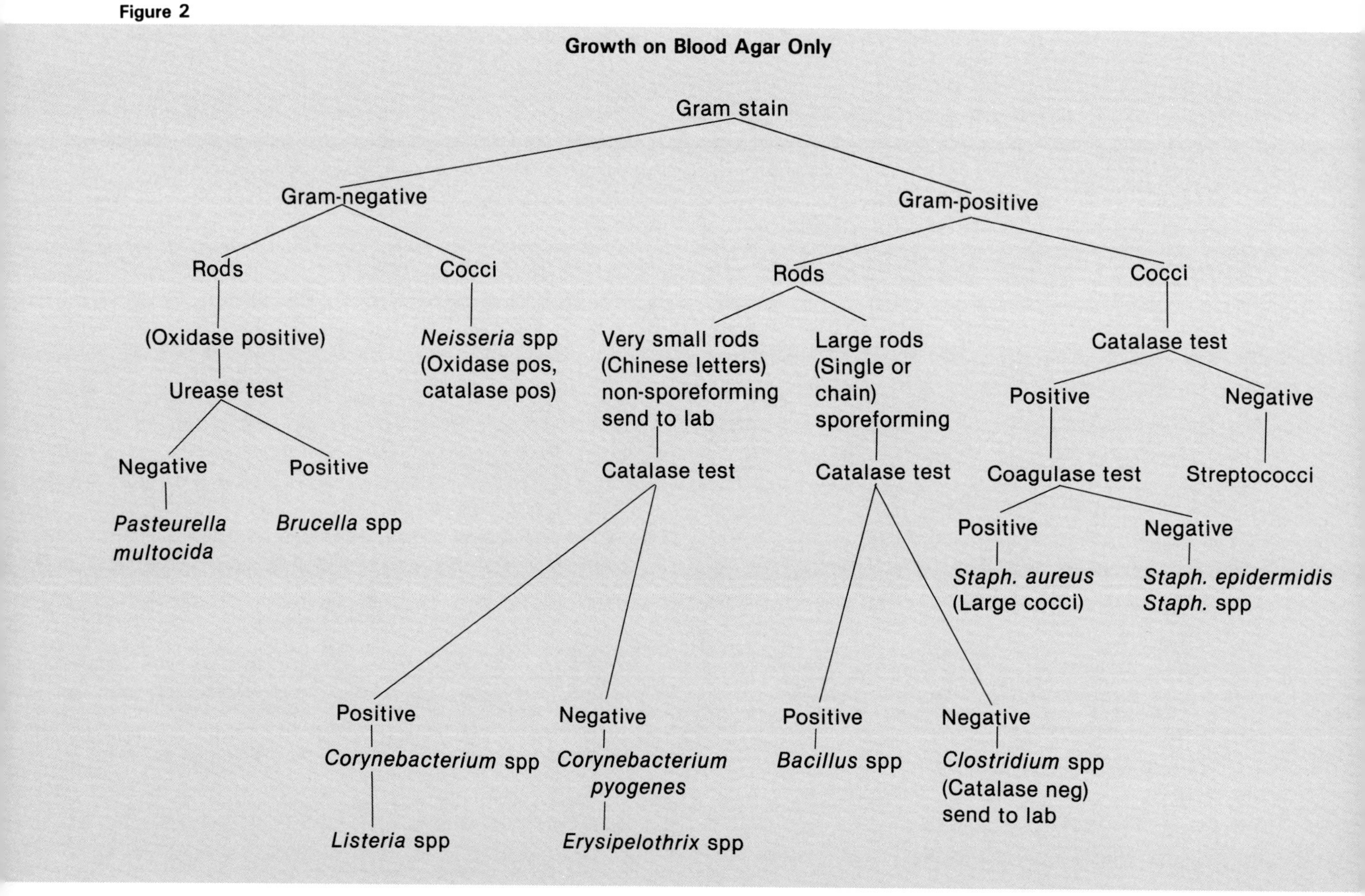

TABLE 2—Microbial Agents Commonly Involved in Skin Infections

Staphylococcus spp
Pseudomonas spp
Various dermatophytes
Various papovaviruses

TABLE 3—Microbial Agents Commonly Involved in Abscess Formation

Staphylococcus spp	*Nocardia asteroides*
Pasteurella spp	Certain fungal agents
Pseudomonas spp	*Blastomyces dermatitidis*
Streptococcus spp	*Crytococcus neoformans*

TABLE 5—Bacteria Commonly Involved in Ear Infections

Pseudomonas spp	*Staphylococcus* spp
Proteus spp	*Klebsiella* spp

TABLE 6—Bacteria Commonly Involved in Vaginal Infections

Brucella spp	*Pseudomonas* spp
Staphylococcus spp	*Pasteurella* spp
Streptococcus spp	

Figure 3

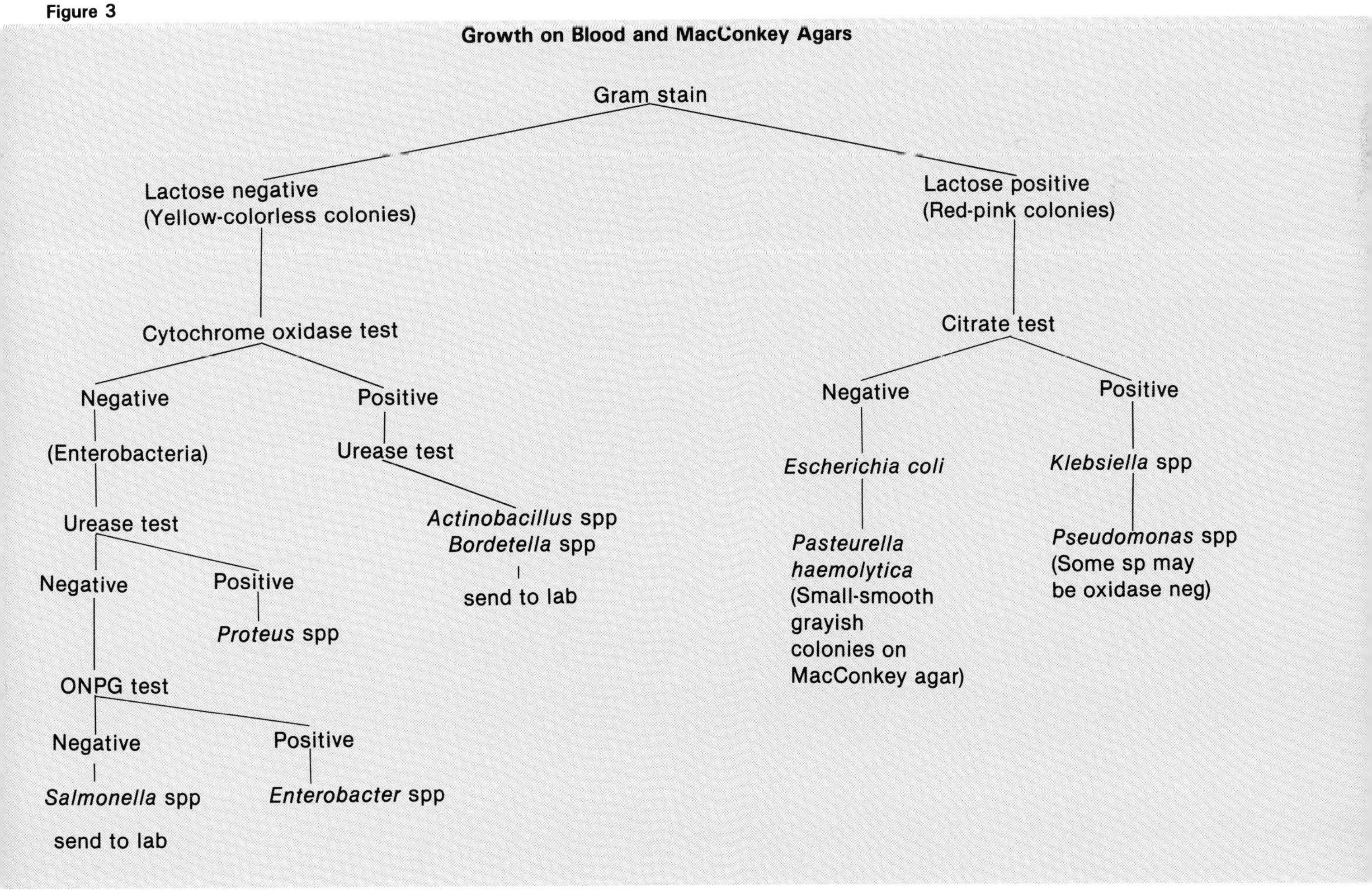

needed. Potassium hydroxide can be used if the Gram stain is inconclusive in determining a Gram-positive or Gram-negative organism. In addition, Gram-negative organisms tend to produce large colonies on blood agar, whereas Gram-positive bacteria produce smaller colonies.

Hemolysis on blood agar plates often indicates the presence of a pathogenic organism. Yeast organisms require about 48 hours to grow and require Gram staining for identification.

Figures 2 and 3 are flow charts useful in differentiating certain organisms that grow only on blood agar or on blood and MacConkey agar. Gram-positive organisms encountered most frequently include Staphylococcus and Streptococcus species. *Staphylococcus* spp are differentiated from *Streptococcus* spp by their positive catalase reaction (*Figure 2*). *Corynebacterium* is a third Gram-positive genus that may be encountered in clinical microbiology. These organisms are seen as club-shaped or pleomophic rods. Remember, pathogens usually grow to pure culture; or are the predominate colonies on a plate; thus, scanty growth should be disregraded.

Gram-negative organisms that are not identified with flow charts (*Figures 2* & *3*) may be identified by one of the commercial systems.

a) Micro ID® (General Diagnostics)

b) API® (Analytab Products)

Each distinct group of colonies found on blood and MacConkey agar plates should be streaked on a Mueller-Hinton plate for sensitivity studies. One to two drops of sterile water help disperse the colonies during the streaking process. On 150 mm Mueller-Hinton plates, 12 antibiotic disks are pressed equally into the agar. The plate is incubated in an inverted position until growth occurs. The results are recorded as *sensitive* or *resistant* depending on growth around each antibiotic disk.

Other test media are available for direct identification and sensitivity of common pathogenic bacteria (Bactassay™—Pitman-Moore), (Unibac™—Bio-Dynamics). Combination test plates include approximately five different test media that differentiate organisms and develop a sensitivity profile.

Bactassay plates contain Mueller-Hinton agar for antibiotic sensitivity testing, MacConkey agar for identifying Gram-negative bacteria that ferment lactose, brain heart infusion agar to support growth of all common aerobic pathogens encountered in veterinary medicine, mannitol salt agar which is selective for staphylococci, and streptosel agar for selectively growing streptococci.

The advantages of combination plates are the ease with which a practitioner can tentatively identify an organism and obtain a sensitivity report. The disadvantages are the sometimes erractic results and higher cost (approximately $4/plate). Combination test plates are recommended for use when one or more aerobic bacteria are involved in an infectious process.

Combination plates are not recommended for use when cultures are taken from anatomic sites with a normal bacterial flora.

These include the upper respiratory tract, mouth, throat, vagina, and intestine (feces).

Several references are recommended for additional reading.[1,2]

REFERENCES

1. Carter, G.R.: *Essentials of Veterinary Bacteriology and Mycology*. Michigan State Press, East Lansing, Mich., 1976.
2. Coles, B.: Simplified Bacteriology for Veterinary Clinics. *VM/SAC* 77 (5):731-736; 1982.

Figure 4—Test and Reagent Materials

1) Catalase test - identifies the enzyme catalase which attacks peroxidases.
Reagent: 3% Hydrogen peroxide.
Method: Place a colony on slide and add a drop of 3% hydrogen peroxide.
Reaction: Positive = bubbling off of oxygen.
Negative = no change.

2) Oxidase test - detects the presence of the cytochrome oxidase system which is involved in aerobic respiration and permits hydrogen peroxide production.
Reagent: Taxo N® disks (Becton-Dickinson).
Method: Moisten disk with sterile water and place on a colony. Incubate plate for 20 to 30 minutes at 37 centigrade.
Reaction: Positive = black-purple color.
Negative = no color change.

3) Potassium hydroxide (KOH) test - differentiates Gram-positive from Gram-negative organisms.
Reagent: 3% potassium hydroxide.
Method: Place 2 loopfuls of 3% KOH on one large colony.
Reaction: Positive = will either clump or form a uniform suspension.
Negative = will form a viscous solution which strings out when teased with a loop.

4) Coagulase test
Reagent: EDTA fresh plasma (less than 24 hours old) from any species.
Method: Emulsify a large number of colonies into a suspension. Mix a small amount of plasma into the suspension.
Reaction: Positive = white clumps within 5 to 20 seconds.
Negative = No reaction within 3 to 4 minutes.

5) Urease test - certain bacteria contain urease which splits urea into ammonium ions causing an alkaline reaction.
Reagent: Urea disks.
Method: Moisten disk with sterile water and place on a colony. Incubate for 20 to 30 minutes at 37 centigrade.
Reaction: Positive = disk will turn red within 10 minutes.

6) ONPG test - identify late lactose fermenters primarily to differentiate *Enterobacter* from *Salmonella*.
Reagent: ONPG disk.
Method: Same as oxidase and urease tests.
Reaction: Positive = yellow color within 10 to 60 minutes.
Negative = no change.

---

7) Citrate test - further separates lactose positive bacteria and *Pseudomonas* spp from *Pasteurella haemolytica.* Catabolism of citrate produces an alkaline reaction turning bromthymol blue from green to blue.
Reagent: Citrate disks.
Method: Same as oxidase, urease, and ONPG.
Reaction: Positive = green-to-blue color change.
Negative = No change in color.

CHAPTER 34

Veterinary mycology

PATHOGENIC MYCOSES of importance to veterinarians include the superficial mycoses (dermatophytes), which affect only the skin, and the deep mycoses, which are systemically invasive and usually affect the skin only after systemic dissemination.

Superficial mycosis (dermatophytosis)

Microsporum canis, *M. gypseum*, and *Trichophyton mentagrophytes* cause 99% of all clinical cases of dermatophytosis in companion animals in the United States.[1-3] *Microsporum canis* alone causes 98% of all feline cases and 70% of all canine cases.

The incidence of dermatophytosis in companion animals is less than many practitioners think. Reportedly, only 2.12% of all dermatologic problems of small animals are caused by dermatophytes.[2] The incidence of dermatophytosis is greater among young animals (particularly those younger than 3 years) than in older ones. Immunosuppressive drugs such as corticosteroids increase the incidence and severity of the disease process.

Dermatophytic infection is transmitted by direct contact between the skin of susceptible animals and infected hair or scales. The incubation period is at least two weeks. Most animals naturally resist infection. Dermatophytes grow only on hairs that are actively growing (anagen phase). When hair growth stops (telogen phase), fungal growth is arrested. The infection then is established in the epithelium around hair follicles.

During growth, the fungi release metabolic products that cause an inflammatory reaction in the hair follicle. Because this reaction is detrimental to the growth of fungi, the organisms spread to adjacent hair follicles. This circular pattern of spreading leaves a lesion with a healing center and an erythematous periphery. The typical appearance of this lesion gave rise to the term *ringworm* for describing dermatophytic infections. The growth of the fungus causes the hair shaft to break off and the keratin layer of the skin to thicken, resulting in typical focal alopecia and scaling of the skin. If bacteria become trapped in an infected hair follicle, secondary bacterial folliculitis results. For this reason, treatment for dermatophytosis should routinely include appropriate antibiotics.

During its growth phase, *M. canis* can break down keratin and produce a tryptophan metabolite that has a greenish-yellow fluorescence when exposed to an ultraviolet Wood light. *Microsporum gypseum* and *T. mentagrophytes* will not fluoresce under a Wood light. All three of these dermatophytes grow on the outside of the hair shaft (ectothrix). Tiny fungal arthrospores are visible under direct microscopic inspection of infected hairs (*Figures 1-3*). Microscopically, cultures of the dermatophytes show macroaleuriospores, in very small numbers for *T. mentagrophytes*, in fair numbers for *M. canis* (*Figure 4*), and in enormous numbers for *M. gypseum* (*Figure 5*).

Dermatophytosis involving the toenails and nail beds is called *onychomycosis*. It is most commonly caused by *T. mentagrophytes*. The infection results in misshapen, brittle toenails, a tender nail bed, and pain in the feet.

Diagnosis of dermatophytosis

Dermatophytosis is commonly diagnosed using direct microscopic examination, Wood light examination, or fungal culture.

Direct microscopic examination

Hair and skin scales are removed from the periphery of lesions, placed on a microscopic slide, and cleared with 10% potassium hydroxide in glycerol. Next, a large drop of this solution is deposited on the hair and scales, and a coverslip is applied. The slide is heated gently with a match and allowed to sit for 10 to 20 minutes before it is examined. Figures 1, 2, and 3 show the arthrospores of three common species of dermatophytes.

A commercial clearing and staining solution (Dermassay™—Pitman-Moore) is available that contains potassium hydroxide and dimethyl sulfoxide. Except that the slide is not heated and must be examined within 10 minutes, the examination procedure is the same as described above.

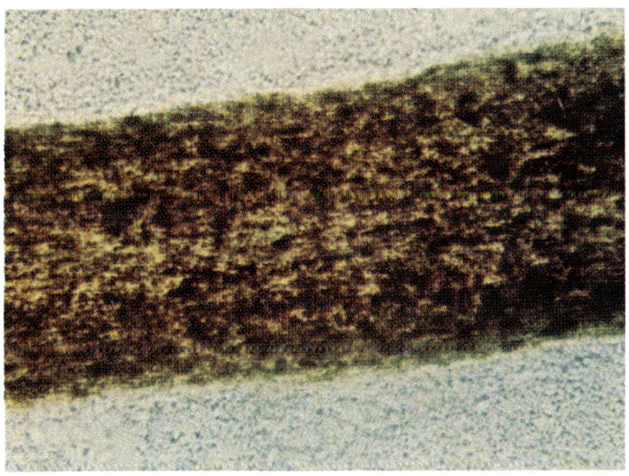

Figure 1—Ectothrix arthrospores of *Microsporum canis.*

Examination by Wood light

This technique aids in diagnosing dermatophytosis caused by *M. canis*. The Wood light is an ultraviolet light of 3600 A wavelength that is filtered through nickel oxide. Broken hairs from a suspect animal are examined in a dark room. A greenish-yellow fluorescence is considered a positive finding. Care should be taken in interpreting results because some medication, lint, scales, and sebum crusts also fluoresce.

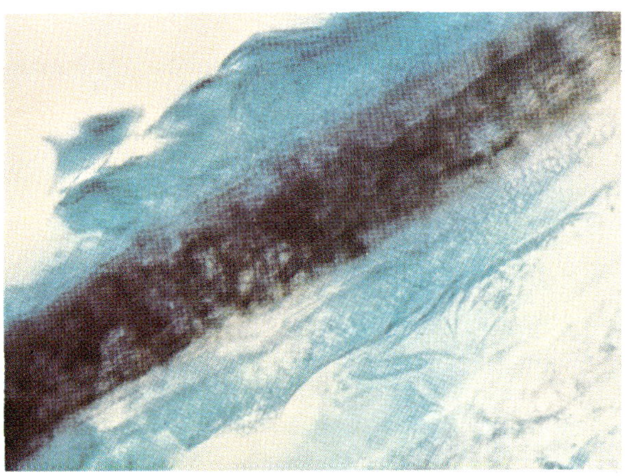

Figure 2—Ectothrix arthrospores of *Microsporum gypseum.*

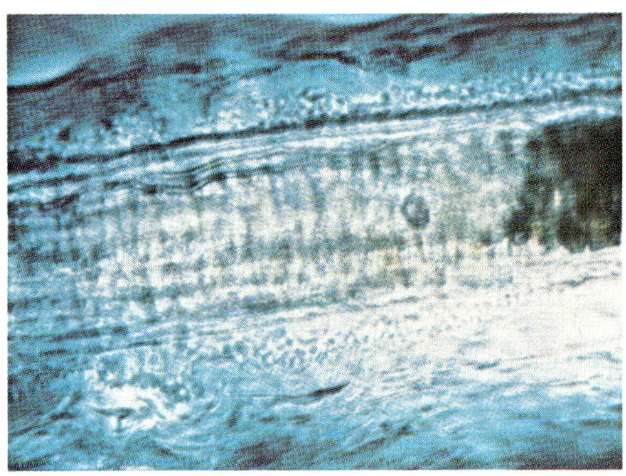

Figure 3—Ectothrix arthrospores of *Trichophyton mentagrophytes.*

Fungal culture

Fungal culture is the most reliable and accurate method of diagnosing dermatophytosis. Although Sabouraud dextrose agar generally is considered the standard medium, it has a major disadvantage for culturing fungi, *i.e.* minimal inhibition of the growth of nonpathogenic fungi. Fungassay™ (Pitman-Moore) is a Sabourand medium containing cycloheximide to inhibit the growth of nonpathogenic fungi, gentamicin plus chlortetracycline to inhibit bacterial growth, and phenol red as a pH indicator. Pathogenic fungi use protein and release alkaline metabolic products that turn the medium red, usually within three to five days. Nonpathogenic fungi that grow despite the presence of cyclohexidine use carbohydrates initially. The protein is used and alkaline metabolic products are released only after the carbohydrates in the medium are exhausted. The nonpathogenic fungi eventually turn the medium red, usually after more than five days.

Specimens of hair, scale, and crust are obtained for culture from the periphery of suspected lesions. The Mackenzie brush technique can be used to identify infected carrier cats that have no apparent lesions. A sterile toothbrush is used to brush the entire coat. Next, the bristles are pressed firmly onto the agar medium, leaving scale and hair debris. The cap is replaced loosely to facilitate the exchange of air during incubation, which is best at room temperature. The culture is identified with the client's name and the date, and is set aside for daily observation.

The organisms grown on the medium are identified by placing a small sample of the fungal colony on a microscope slide. Lactophenol cotton blue stain and a coverslip are applied. The specimen then is examined microscopically for the presence of macroaleuriospores.

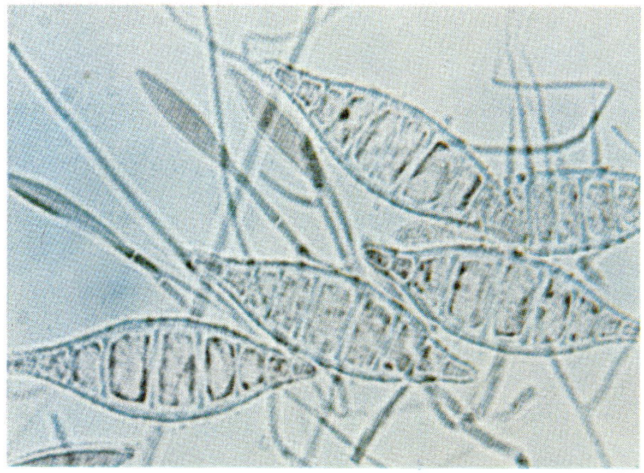

Figure 4—Macroaleuriospores of *Microsporum canis.* The thick-wall spores contain more than six septa.

Treatment of dermatophytosis

Treatment of dermatophytosis is directed toward eliminating infection from the host, preventing further dissemination of infective materials, and removing infective materials already disseminated into the environment. Hair should be clipped from the lesions or, in generalized cases, from the entire body. Bathing the patient weekly with shampoos containing iodine such as Betadine (Purdue Frederick) or Weladol™ (Pitman-Moore) helps prevent further spread of the lesions and dissemination of infective material. Furniture, bedding, and rugs should be vacuumed thoroughly or disinfected with diluted Clorox® . Vacuum-cleaner bags and air-conditioner filters should be discarded.

The primary systemic treatment is griseofulvin in microsize form given daily at a minimum dosage of 20 mg/lb for at least six weeks. Therapy should be continued for at least two weeks after recovery seems apparent. Adding fat in the form of vegetable oil to the patient's diet increases absorption of the drug. An ultramicrosize form of griseofulvin (Gris-Peg® —Dorsey) is more readily absorbed than the microsize form, allowing treatment with one-half the microsize dose. Because it is highly teratogenic, griseofulvin should not be administered to pregnant animals. It also can cause nausea when given on an empty stomach.

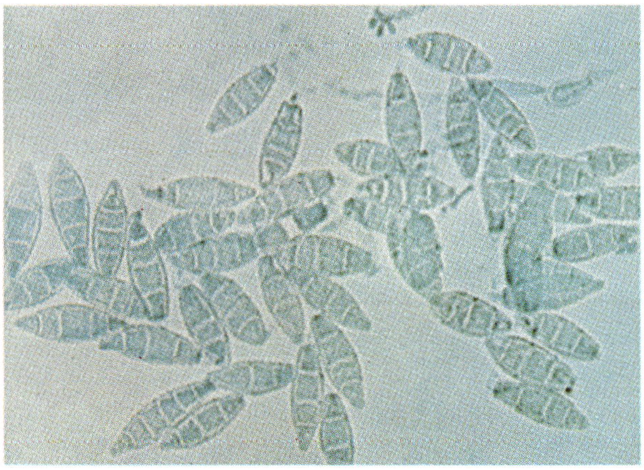

Figure 5—Macroaleuriospores of *Microsporum gypseum.* Note the thin-walled, pointed ends with two or three septa.

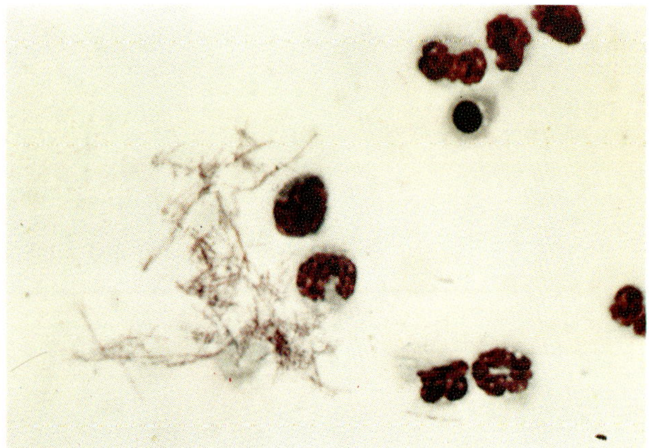

Figure 6—*Nocardia asteroides:* beaded filamentous rods from the pleural fluid of a dog affected with systemic nocardiosis.

Treatment of onychomycosis can require many months of continous therapy. The broad-spectrum, topical, local fungicidal agents such as miconazole, cuprimyxin, and thiobendazole are effective, especially when used in conjunction with griseofulvin.

Deep mycoses

Deep mycoses include those that affect subcutaneous tissue and those that are systemically invasive.

Subcutaneous mycoses

The subcutaneous mycoses, which usually enter the body through a wound in the skin, tend to remain localized and spread regionally via the lymphatic system. Most of these organisms are saprophytes found in the soil. They produce infection only in conjunction with immunodeficiency, prolonged antibiotic or corticosteroid therapy, or debilitating disease. The hallmark of these infections is the presence of chronic, ulcerative, pyogranuloma lesions that do not respond to routine therapy. The common subcutaneous mycoses are 1) sporotrichosis, 2) phycomycosis, 3) mycetoma, 4) aspergillosis, and 5) phaeohyphomycosis.

Sporotrichosis, caused by *Sporotrichum schenckii*, produces nodules and ulcers, usually associated with the lymphatics. When disseminated systemically, it infects mainly the lungs and liver. Diagnosis is best made by culture. Treatment is 20% sodium iodide at a dose of 22 mg/lb for dogs and 11 mg/lb for cats. Cats are sensitive to iodine compounds; signs of toxicity are vomiting, depression, anorexia, and hypothermia.

Treatment for the disseminated form of the disease includes amphotericin B (Fungizone® —Squibb) given at a dosage of 0.25 mg/kg three days per week in 150 to 500 ml of 5% dextrose and water. Because amphotericin B is nephrotoxic, the blood urea nitrogen (BUN) level should be determined before each treatment. If the BUN rises to 60 mg/dl or more, the dosage should be reduced or discontinued.

Ketoconazole (Nizoral® —Janssen) is a new oral systemic antifungal agent. The usual dose of 15 mg/lb/day appears to be effective and to cause few side effects.

Phycomycosis (mucormycosis) is caused by phycomycetes such as *Mucor*, *Rhizopus*, *Absidia*, and *Hyphomyces* spp. Visceral and subcutaneous forms

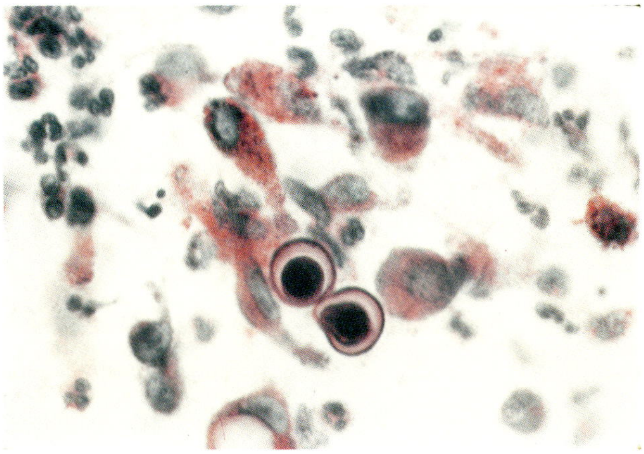

Figure 7—*Blastomyces dermatitidis:* budding yeast organisms with double-contoured walls from a patient with systemic blastomycosis.

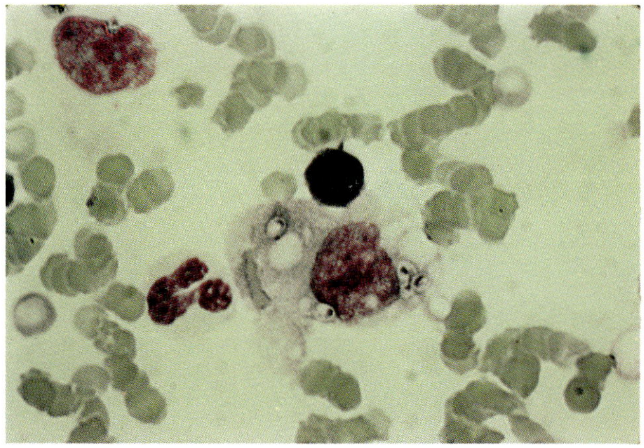

Figure 8—*Histoplasma capsulatum:* oval, yeast organisms within a phagocyte from the bone marrow of a dog with systemic histoplasmosis.

exist. The disease is treated with amphotericin B.

Mycetoma is caused by *Actinomyces*, *Nocardia*, *Curvularia*, *Allescheria*, and *Madurella* species of fungi. They usually cause granulomatous lesions that are best treated by surgical excision. If *Actinomyces* or *Nocardia* infection becomes systemic (*Figure 6*), ampicillin combined with trimethoprim and sulfadiazine is given at the usual dosage.

Aspergillosis is primarily a respiratory infection seen most often in birds. In companion animals, it can present as chronic rhinitis/sinusitis. Diagnosis can be made on results of culture, histopathology, or serology. The prognosis is poor, and treatment is seldom effective.

Phaeohyphomycosis, a subcutaneous infection caused by *Dreschlera spicifera*, has been known to occur only in horses, cats, and man. The lesions are subcutaneous nodules that develop into draining fistulous tracts. Treatment involves surgical excision. The infection rarely disseminates.

Systemic mycoses

The systemic mycoses include coccidioidomycosis, blastomycosis, histoplasmosis, and cryptococcosis. Except for cryptococcosis, these diseases are seen more often in dogs than cats. Infection usually is acquired by inhalation, and the initial disease process is either a sinusitis or pneumonia. The diseases may disseminate to lymph nodes and other visceral organs.

Coccidioidomycosis is caused by *Coccidioides immitis*, which is enzootic to southwestern United States and northern Mexico. Diagnosis is confirmed by a precipitin and complement-fixation test developed specifically for veterinary use. Treatment is with amphotericin B or ketoconazole.

Blastomycosis, caused by *Blastomyces dermatitidis*, is enzootic to the eastern United States and southern Canada. Figure 7 shows the typical thick-wall budding yeast with its double-contoured walls. The lesions are pyogranulomatous and suppurative. Diagnosis is by serology, and treatment is the same as for other systemic fungal infections.

Histoplasmosis, caused by *Histoplasma capsulatum*, is distributed worldwide. Clinical signs include chronic cough, gradual weight loss, diarrhea, and pyrexia. Diagnosis is by serology and demonstration of the oval yeast bodies in reticuloendo-

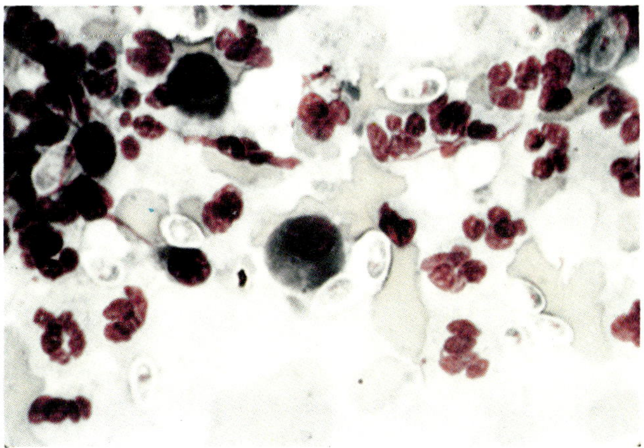

Figure 9—*Cryptococcus neoformans:* small yeast cells surrounded by a gelatinous capsule from nasal exudate of a cat with cryptococcosis.

thelial cells (*Figure 8*).

Cryptococcosis is caused by *Cryptococcus neoformans* and spread most commonly in bird droppings. In cats, it frequently is manifested as a refractory sinusitis. Diagnosis is by serology or demonstration of the small, round, yeast cells surrounded by a large gelatinous capsule (*Figure 9*). Treatment is the same as for other systemic mycoses.

ACKNOWLEDGMENT

The authors thank the editors of Medical Mycology, a Scope® publication by Upjohn, for permission to reprint Figures 1 through 5.

REFERENCES

1. Blakemore, J.C.: Dermatophyte Test Medium. *VM/SAC 66*:357-359; 1971.
2. Blakemore, J.C.: Dermatomycosis. In *Current Veterinary Therapy-V* (R.W. Kirk, ed.). W.B. Saunders, Philadelphia, Pa., 1974; pp 422-437.
3. Muller, G.H.; Kirk, R.W.: Cutaneous Mycology. In *Small Animal Dermatology*. W.B. Saunders, Philadelphia, Pa., 1976; pp 270-295.

10 Miscellaneous

CHAPTER 35

Water, electrolyte, and acid/base balance

In healthy animals, water metabolism and electrolyte and acid/base balances are precisely controlled physiologically to maintain normal homeostasis. Minor alterations in this balance can lead to serious consequences, including death. Therapeutic management of most disease processes that are serious enough to warrant hospitalizing the patient require evaluation of the animal's water balance and, frequently, the electrolyte and acid/base balance. The most common causes of fluid and electrolyte disturbances are loss of gastrointestinal secretions resulting from vomiting and/or diarrhea, failure of conservation by the renal system, or inadequate exogenous intake.

Water balance

Water constitutes 60% of an animal's body weight. Approximately 25% of this water is extracellular, including interstitial and intravascular fluids. The remaining 35% is intracellular fluid. Only the volume of extracellular water is directly regulated. This is done primarily by the kidneys, which conserve water by retaining sodium and producing a smaller volume of more-concentrated urine when the volume of extracellular fluid is less than normal. When the volume of extracellular fluid is greater than normal, the kidneys eliminate a larger volume of more-dilute urine.

Although the renal mechanism of water control is efficient, it must work concurrently with a thirst mechanism mediated by a functional central nervous system. Polydipsia, which occurs when the thirst mechanism is overstimulated, is defined as water intake greater than 50 ml/lb/day. Polyuria, which occurs when the renal mechanism is maximally stimulated to eliminate fluid overload, is defined as urine output exceeding 25 ml/lb/day.

Fluid deficit can be estimated on the basis of clinical and laboratory data and is usually expressed as percent dehydration. This percentage can be estimated by means of physical examination. The degree of skin turgor or decreased elasticity is determined by pinching the skin and observing the time required for it to return to its normal flat state. Skin turgor should be checked in the lumbar region because the skin of the neck is less elastic and pinching it can provide misleading results. Additionally, the skin of old or cachetic animals becomes less elastic, making estimation of dehydration in these animals more difficult.

Dehydration can become apparent when about 5% of the body weight is lost. Skin turgor is then slightly less than normal, and the mouth is dry. Loss of 8% of body weight represents moderate loss of fluids, and pinched lumbar skin slowly returns to normal. The pulse may be weak and the animal depressed. Loss of 10% of body weight is serious; the skin loses its elasticity, the eyes sink into the orbits, and signs of hypovolemic shock may be present. Loss of 12% or more body weight is life-threatening.

Some laboratory tests also indicate dehydration: elevated packed cell volume, hemoglobin, total protein, and increased urine specific gravity. The amount of fluid needed to replace the deficit can be calculated by the formula:

Percent dehydration × body weight (lb) × 500 ml = total body deficit (ml).

This amount of fluids plus the normal amount

lost daily (usually about 25 to 30 ml/lb/day) plus the estimated loss from vomiting, diarrhea, etc., should be given over a 24-hour period. In cases of severe hypovolemic shock, fluids can be given much more rapidly. Experimentally, as much as 45 ml/lb has been given during the first hour to healthy dogs, without adverse effects.[1]

The specific types of fluids needed for replacement and maintenance depend on the electrolyte and acid/base balance. If the specific values for electrolyte and acid/base are known, the selection of appropriate fluids is relatively easy. Often, though, these values cannot be obtained in clinical practice. In those instances, clinical judgment, based on knowledge of the disease process and route of fluid loss (*i.e.* vomiting, diarrhea), dictates the selection of replacement fluids.

Types of fluids

Polyionic solutions

These fluids contain multiple electrolytes and water in a concentration closely resembling that of extracellular fluid. Lactated Ringer solution, the most common, contains physiologic concentrations of sodium (Na^+), chloride (Cl^-), calcium (Ca^{++}) and potassium (K^+) together with 28 mEq of lactate/liter. The lactate is metabolized into bicarbonate ion (HCO_3^-).

Lactated Ringer solution is most often the fluid of choice for replacing deficits of extracellular fluid. It is isotonic (*i.e.* osmotically balanced with the normal extracellular fluid). Ringer solution is the same as lactated Ringer solution except it lacks the lactate. It is most useful for correcting dehydration associated with systemic alkalosis brought on by profound vomiting. When needed, additional electrolyte solutions such as potassium chloride (KCl) can be added to these polyionic solutions.

Saline solutions

These contain water and sodium chloride (NaCl). Isotonic saline solution, containing 0.9% NaCl, is most commonly used. Hypertonic saline solutions that contain 5% saline are available; they are used primarily for dialysis. Hypotonic saline solution (0.45%) is also available; it is useful in treating for hypernatremia and replacing deficits where mostly water but no electrolytes are lost.

Dextrose solutions

Water and dextrose in varying percentages make up these solutions. The one closest to isotonic and most frequently used is 5% dextrose. Because dextrose is rapidly metabolized to carbon dioxide and water, it is almost equivalent to free water. Hypertonic solutions of dextrose (20% and 50%) are used to correct hypoglycemia and to provide calories in parenteral nutrition. Each gram of dextrose supplies 4 Kcal of energy. Dextrose solutions are also available in combination with saline and polyionic solutions. These combinations are hypertonic and must be given intravenously.

Mannitol solutions

Mannitol in water is available in 10% and 20% concentrations. These solutions are hypertonic and must be given intravenously. They are used primarily to induce diuresis and to reduce edema of the central nervous system.

Amino acid solutions

Amino acids and water are available in concentrations of 3.5%, 5%, 7.5%, 8%, and 10% (Travasol® —Travenol). They are used for parenteral nutrition, are extremely hypertonic and must be given slowly via the intravenous route. The preferred method of administration is through a long indwelling catheter (Venocath® —Abbott), into a large central vein.

Fat emulsion solutions

Fat emulsion solutions contain fatty acids and are available in 10% solution (Intralipid® —Cutter). They are used in parenteral nutrition, usually combined with amino acid solutions and dextrose. They are given slowly into a large central vein.[2]

Potassium chloride

This electrolyte is available in 20-ml and 50-ml ampules containing 2 mEq/ml of potassium. It is used to supplement other fluids in cases of hypokalemia. The potassium is added at a rate of 10 to 60 mEq/L of solution and given at a rate no faster than 0.25 mEq/lb/hour.

Sodium bicarbonate

Supplied in ampules and 100-ml bottles containing roughly 1 mEq of HCO_3^-/ml, it is used to reduce acidosis. It can be given slowly, intravenously or mixed with intravenous fluids. Sodium bicarbonate can form insoluble calcium carbonate when added to fluids containing calcium. When this solution is given, care should be taken not to overload the patient with sodium ions.

Calcium gluconate

This solution is supplied in ampules containing 10% calcium. It is used intravenously to correct hypocalcemic tetany, and intracardially in cases of cardiac arrest. When needed, it can be added to other fluids in cases of hypocalcemia.

Electrolyte balance

The most clinically important electrolytes are sodium, potassium, chloride, and bicarbonate. Sodium and potassium are usually assayed by flame photometry. The initial cost of instrumentation is relatively high, but operation and maintenance are simple and the cost per test is low. An excellent flame photometer is the IL 343 (Instrumentation Laboratories). Bicarbonate and chloride assays can be inexpensively done with an Oxford Titrator (Oxford Laboratories). This instrument can also be used to assay calcium and magnesium.

Sodium and potassium

The normal serum sodium value for dogs is 143 ± 6 mEq/L; for cats 151 ± 6 mEq/liter. When the value is less than normal the condition is called *hyponatremia*; when the value is greater than normal the condition is referred to as *hypernatremia*. The normal serum potassium value for dogs is 4.4 to 5.7 mEq/L; for cats 4.0 to 5.0 mEq/liter. *Hypokalemia* designates levels below normal, and *hyperkalemia* designates levels above normal.

Hyponatremia is seen in anorectic patients that drink a large amount of water but lose water and electrolytes through vomiting or diarrhea. It is also seen classically in combination with hyperkalemia in patients with Addison disease. Many practitioners consider a sodium-to-potassium ratio of 23:1 or less to be diagnostic for Addison disease. Hyponatremia is often produced iatrogenically by low-salt diets and by diuretic therapy used in managing congestive heart failure. Correction of hyponatremia is best accomplished with 0.9% saline solution. Hypertonic saline solutions should be used only in serious cases and in hospitals in which the sodium level can be closely monitored.

Hypernatremia often occurs with dehydration resulting from vomiting, fever, and hyperventilation; from excessive exogenous intake (salt poisoning); and from water restriction—especially in the presence of diabetes mellitus and diabetes insipidus. Hypernatremia indicates intracellular dehydration and is frequently associated with hypokalemia. The hypokalemia is a greater threat to survival than is hypernatremia. Hypernatremia is best treated by intravenous administration of 2½% dextrose in one-half strength lactate Ringer's.

Administration of glucose solutions to hypokalemic animals further reduces the extracellular potassium level by promoting potassium transfer into the body cells. For this reason, dextrose solutions should not be used unless the potassium value is normal. Dehydrated patients cannot be assumed to be hypernatremic. If the dehydrated patient happens to be hyponatremic or hypokalemic, the administration of dextrose solutions could cause water toxicity and intensify the hypokalemia. Unless the electrolyte status is known, giving dextrose solutions to dehydrated animals is usually risky.

Hypokalemia accompanies vomiting, diarrhea, diuretic therapy, diabetic ketoacidosis, and respiratory acidosis. Because most of the total body potassium is intracellular, the serum concentration can be used only as a rough guideline. Hypokalemia causes hypotension and depletes potassium in the muscles; it is characterized by weakness.

Potassium deficits can be best restored with lactated Ringer solution supplemented with potassium chloride (10 to 60 mEq/L) and given no faster than 0.25 mEq of potassium/lb/hour. Oral replacement of potassium is possible if the animal is not vomiting; however, care must be taken not to overdose because the oral forms are rapidly and completely absorbed by the small intestine. Serum potassium can be monitored accurately with flame photometry, or roughly with electrocardiography by watching for signs of hyperkalemia (*i.e.*, progressive increasing amplitude [peaking] of the T waves).

Hyperkalemia can result from renal failure, acidosis, low-sodium diet, Addison disease, urinary obstruction, and excess exogenous intake. A classic example of a hyperkalemic crisis is the semicomatose, dehydrated male cat with urinary obstruction. A potassium value of 8 mEq/L or more is associated with life-threatening cardiac arrythmias.

In treating hyperkalemia, the most important assessment is the degree of renal function and/or the presence of obstructive uropathy. If renal function is normal, hyperkalemia can be treated with 5% dextrose, intravenously, to promote diuresis and movement of potassium intracellularly. Sodium bicarbonate also promotes the movement of potassium into the cells by exchange of potassium ion for hydrogen ions, which are then excreted renally.

In cases of severe hyperkalemia, when renal function cannot reduce the potassium concentration, 40 to 50 mEq of sodium bicarbonate and 10 units of regular insulin may be added to a liter of 5% or 10% dextrose in 0.9% saline solution and given intravenously. This treatment drives as much of the potassium as possible into the cells and reduces the extracellular level. The cardiotoxic effects of hyperkalemia can be treated with calcium gluconate given intravenously at an initial dosage of 10 mg/lb, then to effect while the ECG is monitored. Because this procedure does not reduce the amount of potassium in the extracellular fluid, its effects are only temporary.

Acid/base balance

The chloride, bicarbonate and hydrogen ions, plus the carbon dioxide concentration in the body, are closely regulated. They constitute the acid/base balance and are measured collectively as pH.

The normal amount of chloride in canine serum is 100 to 115 mEq/L; in feline serum it is 110 to 120 mEq/liter. Normal levels of bicarbonate for dogs and cats is 17 to 24 mEq/liter. Alterations of chloride values closely follow those of sodium. This is because the negatively charged chloride ions are distributed passively according to the electrical gradient established by the positively charged sodium ions. Notable exceptions are hypochloremia associated with vomiting and excessive loss of hydrochloric acid, and hyperchloremic metabolic acidosis associated with such conditions as severe diarrhea where loss of bicarbonate ions is excessive and the chloride ions are increased to maintain electroneutrality or cation-anion balance.

pH

The normal pH of dogs and cats is 7.4 ± 0.05. Values less than 7.35 indicate acidosis; values greater than 7.45 indicate alkalosis. Variance in pH between 7.2 and 7.6 is not considered sufficiently critical to warrant specific treatment for the pH; treatment is required only for the primary disease contributing to the acid/base imbalance.[3] Any pH value outside of the range, however, is critical, and specific acidifying or alkalizing agents are required. A pH of less than 7.0 and more than 7.8

generally results in death.

Blood pH can be measured with a pH meter or pH and blood gas analyzers (Instrumentation Laboratories). This is expensive and sophisticated instrumentation, usually available only at large veterinary hospitals or in practices in which critical care is emphasized. Laboratories that deal primarily with human medicine may be of little benefit because the heparinized blood to be analyzed must be processed within a couple of hours after it is collected. Also, data from blood gas analysis are usually needed immediately so that optimal therapy can be started. Other methods of evaluating the acid/base balance in animals are clinical evaluation and the bicarbonate determination.

Clinical evaluation is the more important to most practitioners. It is helpful to know that acidosis accompanies certain types of conditions and that alkalosis accompanies others. Gastroenteritis associated with vomiting usually causes metabolic alkalosis due to excess loss of hydrochloride. Gastroenteritis associated with diarrhea usually causes metabolic acidosis due to excess loss of bicarbonate ion. If vomiting and diarrhea occur concomitantly, they tend to counteract each other, resulting in equal loss of acid and base and fluid components. Shock, whether traumatic, hypovolemic, or endotoxic, usually results in acidosis. Experimentally, mortality is greater among dogs in shock that are given blood in acid citrate dextrose solution if the pH of the solution is not adjusted to 7.8 before adminstration. In companion animals with renal disease, metabolic acidosis usually develops due to failure of the kidney to eliminate the acid products of metabolism. However, if the renal disease causes severe vomiting, alkalosis may develop.

Such respiratory disorders as pneumonias, which inhibit ventilation and prevent carbon dioxide from being exhaled, typically result in respiratory acidosis. Respiratory disorders that result in hyperventilation (*e.g.* nervousness, hyperanxiety, heat exhaustion) cause excess loss of carbon dioxide and result in respiratory alkalosis.

Metabolic acidosis is the most common veterinary acid/base imbalance seen clinically. Therapy includes intravenous fluids supplemented with sodium bicarbonate or lactate. The mEq potencies of sodium bicarbonate and lactate are about the same, but lactate must be metabolized before it is used. In the therapeutic management of disease processes that cause metabolic acidosis, when specific data on the animal's acid/base balance are lacking, slow intravenous administration of small doses of sodium bicarbonate (0.5 mEq/lb body weight) are beneficial.

In the therapeutic management of conditions associated with alkalosis, administration of acidifying salts (*e.g.* 0.9% sodium chloride or Ringer solution) to restore fluid volume will help correct the acid/base imbalance. In the case of severe alkalosis, such as occurs with profound vomiting in dogs with pyloric stenosis, ammonium chloride given intravenously at 1 mEq/lb in sterile water will help control the severe acid/base imbalance until the pyloric obstruction can be relieved.

Bicarbonate values can be readily determined with a relatively inexpensive titrimeter (Oxford Titrator—Oxford Laboratories). This instrument measures the plasma bicarbonate by titrating it against a known amount of acid. Values are read from a dial that displays the bicarbonate level in mEq/liter. With this information and the knowledge that the most normal bicarbonate level is 24 mEq/L, the bicarbonate deficit can be calculated by the formula:

$$\text{Body weight (kg)} \times 0.6 \times (24 - \text{patient's bicarbonate level}) = \text{total deficit (mEq)}.$$

This deficit can be overcome by giving sodium bicarbonate intravenously or intraperitoneally. One gram of sodium bicarbonate equals 12 milliequivalent. Most commercial sodium bicarbonate solutions contain about 1 mEq/milliliter.

REFERENCES

1. Cornelius, L.M. *et al*: Physiologic Effects of Rapid Infusion of Ringer's Lactate Solution into Dogs. *Am. J. Vet. Res. 39*:1185-1190; 1978.
2. Goldston, R.T. *et al*: The Clinical Pathology Laboratory: 26 - Management of Gastrointestinal Problems. *VM/SAC 77*(2):171-173; 1982.
3. Sattler, F.P. *et al* (eds.): *Veterinary Critical Care.* Lea & Febiger, Philadelphia, PA., 1981.

CHAPTER 36

Exfoliative cytology

EXFOLIATIVE CYTOLOGY is the study of the origin, structure, function, and pathology of cells 1) that exfoliate into body fluids, 2) aspirated or scraped from tissue masses or lesions *in vivo*, or 3) imprinted from excised tumors onto a glass slide. Exfoliative cytology is an extension of standard hematologic techniques; it involves use of the same stains that are important in the study of blood and bone marrow.[1,2] Tissue imprints and tissue scraping techniques are used on solid lesions and excised tumors. Tissue aspirations are done in cases where lesions or tumors are deep within the patient's body.

Tissue imprints are made by blotting a clean, freshly cut surface of an excised tumor mass onto a slide. Tissue scraping involves superficially cleaning an open lesion, scraping it gently with a scalpel blade, and spreading the cells onto a glass slide. Tissue scraping is useful for studying dense excised tumors, such as those from connective tissue.

Tissue aspirations are made using a 23- or 25-gauge needle with a 12-cc syringe. Aspiration is done while three or four passes through the mass are made at different angles. To avoid rupturing some of the cells, suction pressure should be released before the needle is removed from the mass. Usually, the sample is small and found only in the hub of the needle. Next, the needle is removed from the syringe, which is filled with air. The syringe is reattached to the needle, and the aspirated air is used to force the sample onto a slide. A second slide is placed perpendicularly to the first, and the two slides are spread apart to create a smear. The danger of neoplastic metastasis during needle aspiration should be kept in mind, but, in our experience, this has been more of a theoretical consideration than a clinical complication.

One of the most important uses of exfoliative cytology is for differentiation of inflammatory and neoplastic processes. With practice, the clinician can identify the specific neoplastic disorder or, in the case of inflammation, the specific causes (*Figures 1-7*).

The vaginal smear is a useful form of exfoliative cytology for evaluating the stages of estrus, as well as inflammatory conditions involving the uterus and vagina. A swab for vaginal cytology is obtained while the animal is restrained in a standing position. The tail is elevated, and the lips of the vulva are cleaned. A vaginal speculum is placed, and a sterile swab moistened with saline solution is passed into the vagina. The vaginal mucosa is swabbed using a gentle rotary motion. Next, the swab is rolled onto a clean glass slide, and the smear is stained.

The make-up of vaginal cells varies with the stages of the estrous cycle (*Figures 8-10*). These stages can be identified by using three criteria to judge cytologic samples: 1) color of fluid, 2) characteristics of epithelial cells, 3) presence (or absence) of neutrophils. Vaginal cytology can also aid in detecting vaginal and/or uterine infection. Cornified epithelial cells associated with clumps of neutrophils are not seen in normal vaginal cytology and, thus, usually indicate infection. The presence of bacteria does not necessarily indicate infection because vaginal smears often contain bacteria.

Body fluids commonly studied by means of exfoliative cytology are abdominal, thoracic, and synovial fluid (*Figures 11-17*). Samples are easily obtained by needle aspiration or through the use of indwelling polypropylene catheters. Fluid samples should be checked for turbidity, color, specific gravity, and protein content. Also, white and red blood cell counts should be done. A centrifuged sample is used

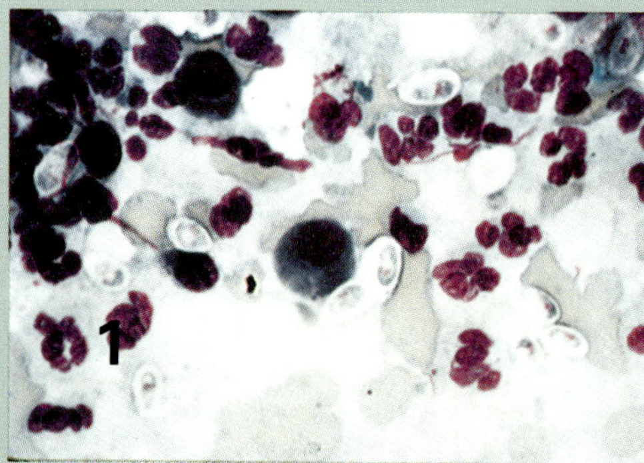

Figures 1 through 7

Differentiation of inflammatory and neoplastic processes.

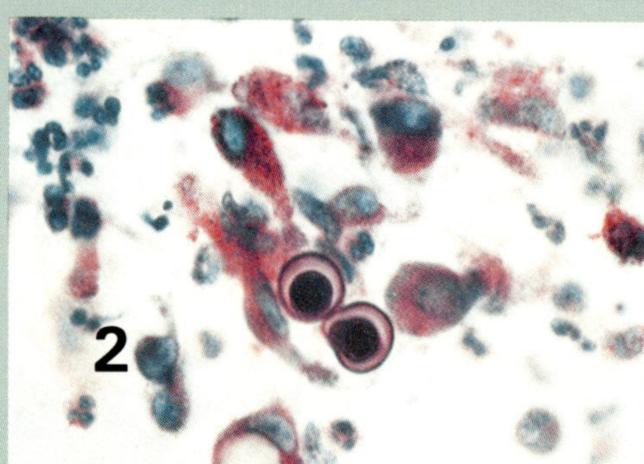

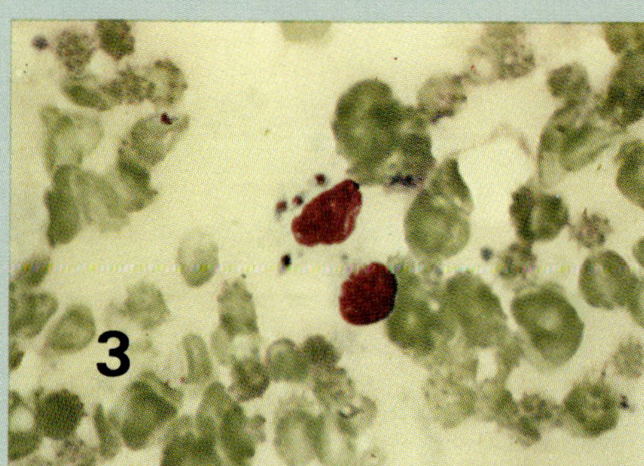

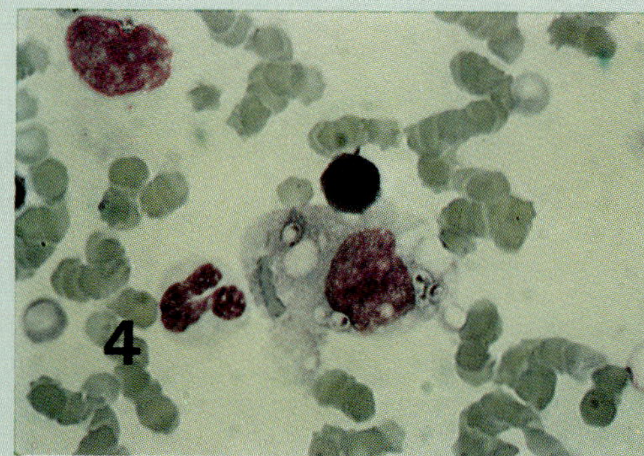

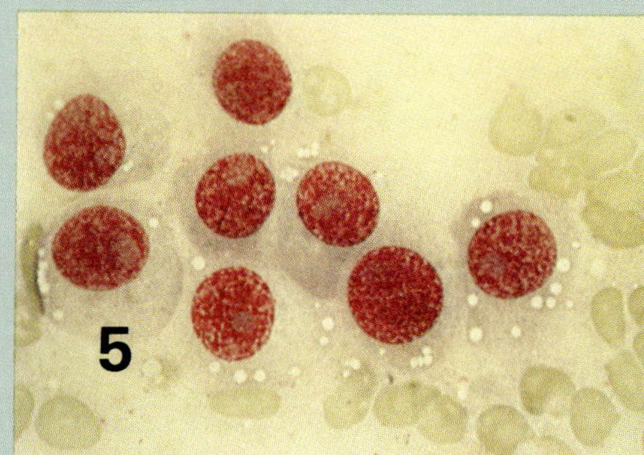

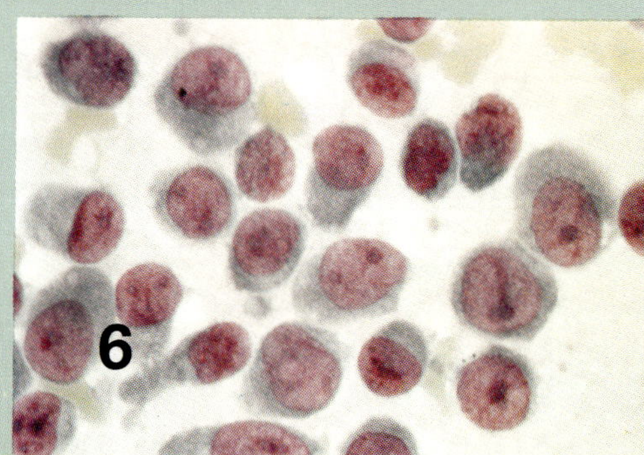

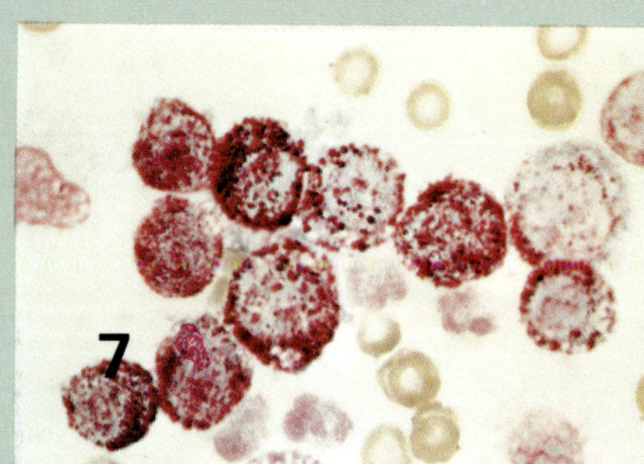

Figure 1—Tissue impression from nasal discharge from a cat affected with unilateral sinusitis. The neutrophils and plasma cells indicate inflammation. The oval-shaped organisms with a clear zone around them are *Cryptococcus.* Thus, the diagnosis is feline cryptococcosis.

Figure 2—Tissue scraping from an ulcerative skin lesion on a dog. Note signs of inflammation, neutrophils, and histiocytes. The large yeast-shaped organisms are *Blastomyces*, indicating a diagnosis of canine blastomycosis.

Figure 3—Tissue imprint from the lung of a dog. The cells are phagocytes, and the banana-shaped organisms with a central nucleus are *Toxoplasma gondii* bodies. The diagnosis is canine toxoplasmosis.

Figure 4—Tissue impression from a specimen of bone marrow taken by biopsy. Note the cells of inflammation, including the large histiocytes that have phagocytized *Histoplasma capsulatum* organisms. The diagnosis is granulomatous osteomyelitis due to histoplasmosis.

Figure 5—Tissue imprint from a nodular tumor on the penis of a dog. The large, uniform group of cells with large nuclei, prominent nucleoli, and abundant cytoplasm indicate neoplasia. The diagnosis is transmissible venereal tumor.

Figure 6—Tissue imprint from a small nodular tumor on the head of a young dog. The large group of uniform cells with large nuclei and prominent nucleoli indicates neoplasia; the diagnosis is histiocytoma. The shape of the tumor mass and its location are important in differentiating this tumor from the transmissible venereal tumor because the cells are similar.

Figure 7—Tissue imprint from a tumor on the scrotum of a dog. The large group of uniformly shaped cells and the absence of inflammatory cells indicate neoplasia. The round nucleus and prominent cytoplasmic granules are characteristic of mast cells. The diagnosis is mast cell tumor.

Figure 8—A vaginal smear done during anestrus is characterized by the presence of mature noncornified epithelial cells and occasional neutrophils and bacterial debris.

Figure 9—Proestrus is characterized by the presence of erythrocytes, neutrophils, and noncornified epithelial cells. Often, if a cotton swab is used to take the smear, erythrocytes won't be on the slide. This is because they are absorbed by the cotton. In such instances, the presence of erythrocytes is best indicated by the reddish color of the cotton swab. The noncornified epithelial cells are large and have oversized nuclei and rounded edges. The chromatin has a vesicular arrangement.

Figure 10—A vaginal smear done during estrus. Note that there are no neutrophils, and the erythrocytes have decreased in number. The cornified epithelial cells are characterized by a pyknotic nucleus and more angular margins to the sides of the cells. Also, the cells fold easily.

All tissue samples were stained with Wright stain.

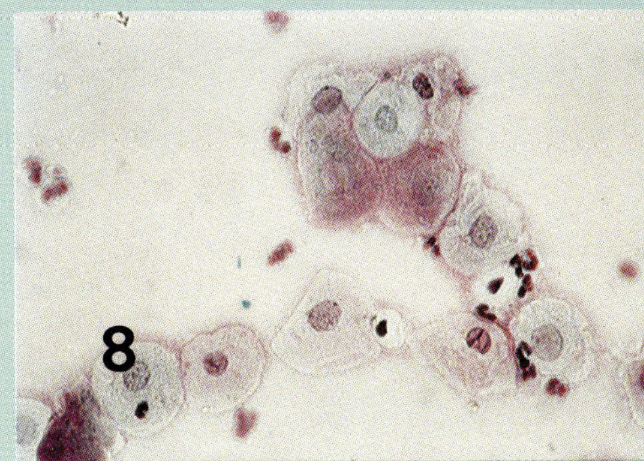

Figures 8 through 10

Make-up of vaginal cells varies with the stages of the estrous cycle.

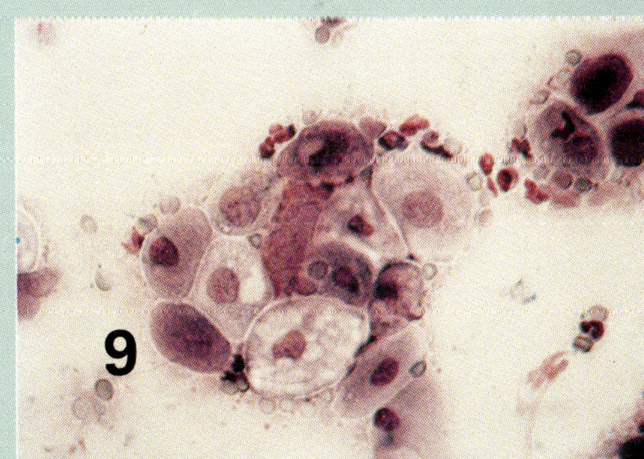

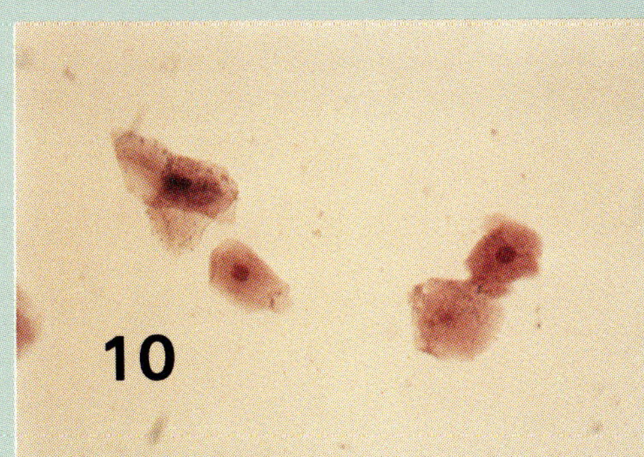

to concentrate cells for cytologic study. It is important to determine whether the fluid is a *transudate* (normal body fluid that accumulates due to altered osmotic pressures) or an *exudate* (fluid that arises as a result of inflammation). Some fluids may or may not be associated with inflammation and are classified as *modified transudates.* Table 1 lists characteristics of these three types of fluids.

Comments

As can easily be seen, cytologic examination of body fluids, tumors, and other lesions can often lead to a specific diagnosis and will almost always enable the clinician to learn whether the cause of the condition is inflammatory or neoplastic. Also, it can usually be determined whether the inflammatory process is acute (neutrophils predominate) or chronic (lymphocytes, plasma cells, and histiocytes predominate). In cases of neoplasia, cytologic examination can usually be used to determine whether the lesion is malignant or benign. Occasionally, the specific cell type (*e.g.* mast cell, lymphoblast) can be ascertained, thus providing a definitive diagnosis.

REFERENCES

1. Seybold, I.M. *et al:* The Basic Clinical Pathology Laboratory-5: Evaluation of the Blood Smear. *VM/SAC* 75(5):781-789; May 1980.
2. Seybold, I.M. *et al:* The Clinical Pathology Laboratory-10: Examination of the Bone Marrow. *VM/SAC* 75(10):1517-1521; October 1980.

TABLE 1—Characteristics of Transudates, Modified Transudates, and Exudates

Determination	Transudate	Modified Transudate	Exudate
Turbidity	Clear	Sometimes slightly turbid	Turbid
Color	Colorless to pale straw	Yellow or red	Variable
Specific gravity	1.018 (or less)	Variable	1.018 (or more)
Total protein	3.0 g/dl (or less)	Variable	3.0 g/dl (or more)
WBC	Low	Low to moderate	Variable to high
RBC	None to few	Variable	Variable
Bacteria/microorganisms	None	None	Variable
Clots	None	None or slight	Frequent
Cells	Few	Variable	Variable to high

Figure 11—Cellular sediment from a sample of thoracic fluid taken from a young dyspneic cat. The uniform grouping of large cells with large nuclei and prominent nucleoli is characteristic of neoplasia. The morphology of the cells is that of lymphoblasts. The diagnosis in this case is feline thymic lymphosarcoma.

Figures 12 & 13—Cells and Sudan-stained fluid from the thorax of a dyspneic cat. The fluid is relatively acellular. Figure 12 shows that the predominant nucleated cell is a small lymphocyte. Figure 13 shows that the fluid stains readily with the fat stain, Sudan III, thus indicating the presence of chyle. The diagnosis is chylothorax.

Figure 14—Sediment of abdominal fluid from a febrile dog. Note the presence of degenerative neutrophils, erythrocytes, and bacteria. These indicate inflammation resulting from bacterial infection. The diagnosis is peritonitis.

Figure 15—Cellular sediment from the thoracic fluid of a dyspneic cat. The principal cells are degenerate neutrophils with intra- and extracellular bacteria. The diagnosis is pyothorax.

Figure 16—Cellular sediment from the thoracic fluid of an older dog. Note that the cells are large, pleomorphic, contain giant nuclei, and are clumped—all criteria of malignancy. At necropsy, the diagnosis was bronchiogenic carcinoma.

Figure 17—Sediment from thoracic fluid from a dyspneic dog. Note that the principal cells are neutrophils. Also present are the beaded, filamentous, rod-shaped bacteria characteristic of *Nocardia.* The diagnosis is nocardiosis.

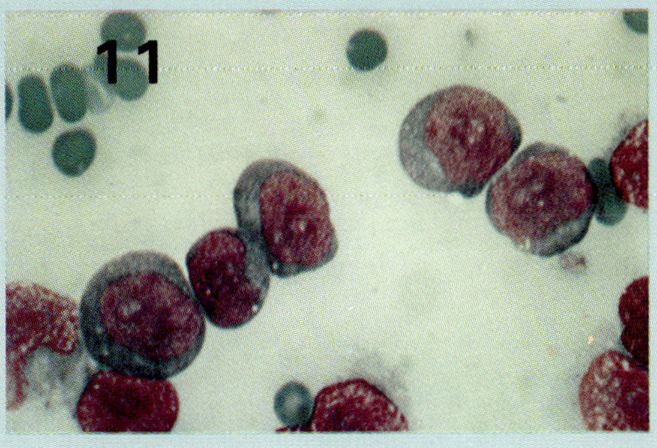

Figures 11 through 17

Abdominal, thoracic, and synovial fluids are studied by means of exfoliative cytology.

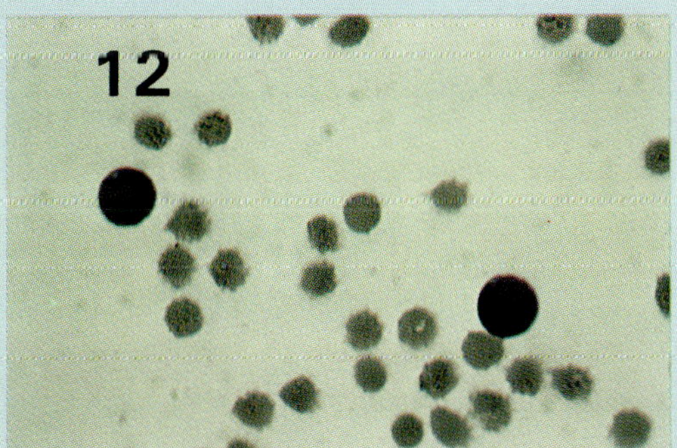

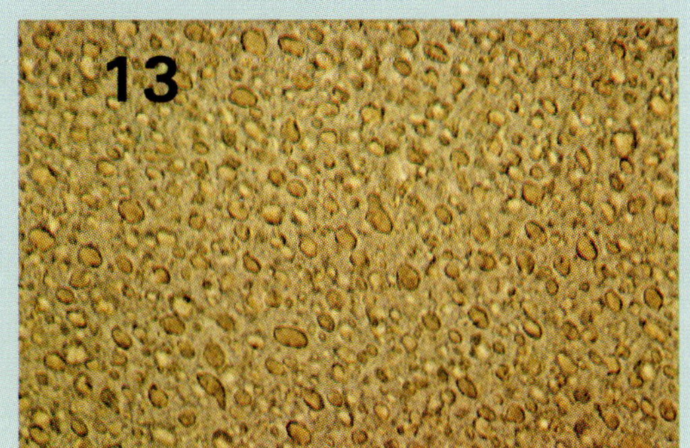

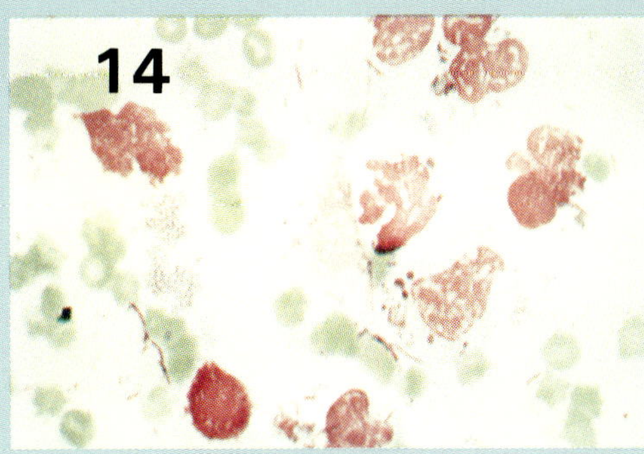

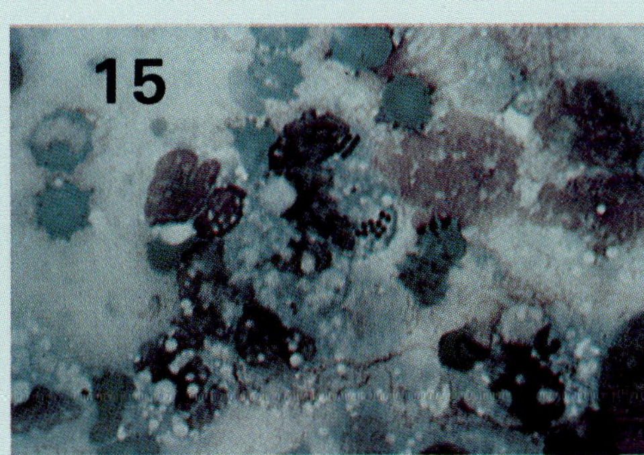

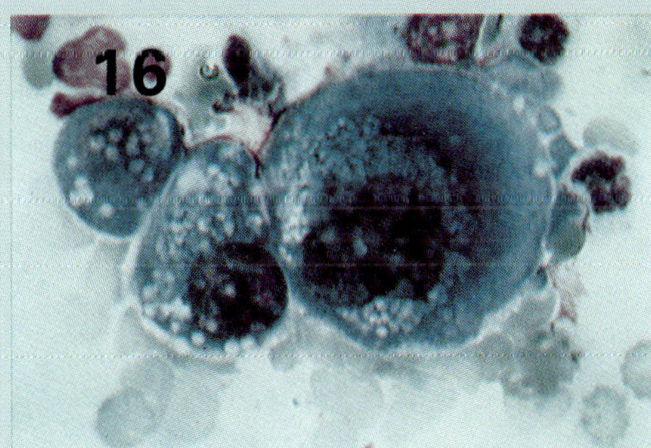

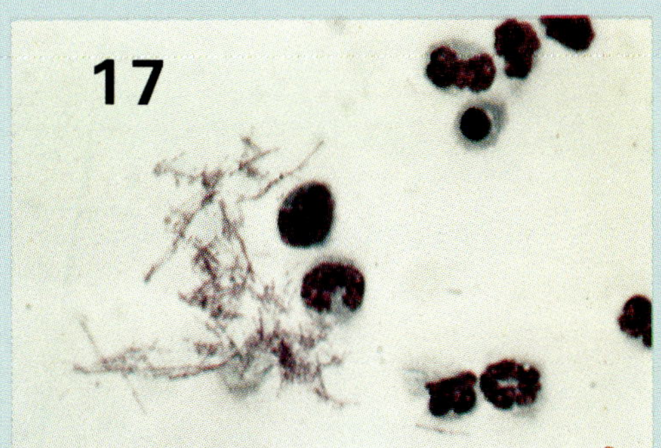

CHAPTER 37

Clinical toxicology

UNTIL RECENTLY, clinical toxicology primarily involved postmortem findings and retrospective investigation. However, as the science of veterinary medicine has matured, many techniques have been developed to aid in diagnosing and treating poisoning cases. The shortness of the diagnostic procedure and the rapidity with which results become available have made clinical toxicology feasible.

A well-equipped clinical toxicology laboratory should have a 1) gas-liquid chromatograph, 2) atomic absorption spectrometer, 3) radiation counter, 4) ultraviolet spectrophotometer, 5) thin-layer chromatographic materials, and 6) ancillary equipment. Personnel should be skilled in operating the equipment and knowledgeable in screening tests for specific signs and history. In addition, quality control is achieved only by routinely performing a certain number of tests. Finally, medicolegal concerns necessitate accurate documented results. Because most veterinary hospitals cannot meet these requirements, toxicology samples probably should be sent to a laboratory.

In most cases of poisoning, the veterinarian first must assimilate the history and results of the physical examination and clinical or toxicologic tests. Then, this material must be interpreted to confirm a diagnosis. Because a multitude of toxicologic tests are available, a screening process must be used in each case to select the proper tests. To ensure accurate laboratory results, the practitioner should exercise care in selecting, processing, and handling specimens for laboratory evaluation.

A complete history including possible poisons, use of pesticides or rodenticides, treatments, habitat, and the weight, age, sex, species, and breed of the animal should be sent with the samples to the laboratory. This information allows the toxicologist to select other tests as needed. Clinical signs, as well as antemortem and postmortem lesions should be included. When dealing with a toxicology laboratory for the first time, it is wise to find out what information is required before submitting samples.

For clinical toxicology, whole blood, serum, plasma, and urine are the preferred samples. Gastric contents can be important in determining whether an animal has had contact with a toxin. But, in most cases, the cause-and-effect relationship between the amount of substance found and its possible toxic effect requires a quantitative measurement from whole blood or one of its fractions.

Specimens should be of adequate size and contain no debris or contaminants. Because most samples are mailed and thus subjected to unknown variables, they should be carefully packaged for shipping. Usually, tissues are frozen, and serum and blood are refrigerated. Each specimen should be placed in a separate glass or plastic container and labeled with the name of the owner and animal, as well as the tissue or specimen.

In cases where histopathology is required, samples in 10% formalin should be forwarded to the laboratory in different containers. (If there is doubt as to whether histopathology specimens are needed, the laboratory should be phoned or both frozen and formalin-fixed specimens should be sent.) Liquid specimens should be placed in leak-proof containers and packed with newspapers or other protective padding. Other specimens can be placed in plastic bags with ice.

Specimens from live animals for toxicologic studies should include: Serum - 5 ml, plasma - 5 ml, whole blood - 10 ml, urine - 50 ml, and bait or vomitus - 200 g. Specimens from dead animals should include: Serum - 5 ml; whole blood - 10 ml; urine - 50 ml; entire brain; and liver, kidney, spleen, body fat - 100 g of each. If possible, 500 g of stomach contents should also be collected. If infection or inflammation is suspected, the brain should be bisected and one half mixed in 10% buffered formalin and the other frozen.

The practitioner should be aware of common causes of poisonings in his or her practice area. Often, on the basis of the history and clinical signs, a tentative diagnosis can be made, therapy initiated, and a realistic prognosis made. The National Pesticide Telecommunications Network* provides information on pesticide toxicities, including the toxic principle and therapy. Table 1 lists poison control centers in the United States. In Table 2, certain poisons and sample(s) required for laboratory confirmation of the diagnosis are presented.

Common causes of toxicity are:

1. Rodenticides
   a. strychnine
   b. monofluoracetate
   c. warfarin
   d. thallium
2. Food intoxications (enterotoxemias)
3. Insecticides
   a. organophosphates
   b. carbamate
   c. chlorinated hydrocarbons
4. Snake venom
5. Arsenic
6. Metaldehyde
7. Fungi
8. Lead and antifreeze
9. Drug reactions or interactions

*Phone toll-free 1-800-845-7633

TABLE 1—Poison Control Centers[1,2] in the United States

Poison Information Center
New York City Department of Health
Bureau of Laboratories
455 First Avenue
New York, NY 10016
Phone: 212-340-4495

The Chicago Master Center
Rush-Presbyterian-St. Luke's Medical Center
1753 West Congress Parkway
Chicago, IL 60612
Phone: 312-942-5969

Poison Control Center
St. Mary of Nazareth Hospital Center
1120 North Leavitt Street
Chicago, IL 60622
Phone: 312-292-5391

Poison Control Center
South Chicago Community Hospital
2320 East 93rd Street
Chicago, IL 60617
Phone: 312-978-2000, ext. 264, 265 or 297

Poison Control Center
W. I. Cook Children's Hospital
1212 West Lancaster Avenue
Fort Worth, TX 76102
Phone: 817-336-5561, ext. 17, or at night 336-5527

Poison Control Center
The Thomas J. Fleming Memorial Center
Children's Hospital of Los Angeles
Post Office Box 54700
4650 Sunset Boulevard
Los Angeles, CA 90054
Phone: 213-664-2121

1. Oehme, F.W.: Laboratory Diagnosis of Chemical Intoxications. In *Vet. Clin. N. Am.*, vol. 6. W.B. Saunders, Philadelphia, PA, p 732.
2. Oehme, F.W.: Use of Laboratories for the Chemical Analysis of Tissues. In *Current Veterinary Therapy-VI.* W.B. Saunders, Philadelphia, PA, pp 101-106.

Comments

The practitioner should not only collect and prepare toxicology specimens but should also work closely with laboratory personnel in evaluating results. Some laboratories have frequent exposure to certain toxins and are competent in obtaining accurate results. However, species variation may cause difficulty in some laboratories, requiring the practitioner to help determine the significance of a test

TABLE 2—Specimens Required for Specific Tests*

Poison or Analysis Requested	Specimen Required	Amount of Specimen Desired	Comments
Ammonia**	Whole blood or serum	5 ml	Frozen (1-2 drops of saturated $HgCl_2$ may be used instead of freezing rumen contents)
	Stomach contents (composite)	100 g	
	Urine	5 ml	
ANTU	Stomach and intestine contents	200 g	Can be detected only within 12 to 24 hours after ingestion
	Liver	200 g	
Arsenic	Liver	50 g	
	Kidney	50 g	
	Feed	100 g	
	Stomach contents	100 g	
	Urine	50 ml	
Calcium	Serum	2 ml	Serum must *not* be hemolyzed; separate clot before transit.
	Feed	25 g	
Carbon monoxide	Whole blood	15 ml	
Chloride	*See* Sodium		
Chlorinated hydrocarbon insecticides	Brain	0.5 cerebrum	Must not be contaminated with hairs or stomach contents; preferable to use chemically clean glass jars; avoid plastic containers.
	Body fat	100 g	
	Stomach contents	100 g	
	Liver	50 g	
	Kidney	50 g	
	Whole blood	10 ml	
Copper	Kidney	50 g	
	Liver	50 g	
	Whole blood or serum	10 ml	
	Feces	100 g	
Cyanide	Whole blood	10 ml	Freeze specimen promptly in air-tight container.
	Liver	50 g	
	Forage, silage	100 g	
	Other materials	100 g	
Ethylene glycol	Serum	10 ml	
	Kidney (in formalin)	Whole organ	One kidney, both in small animals
	Urine	10 ml	
Fluoroacetate	Stomach contents	All available	Frozen
	Kidney	One whole	
	Urine	50 g	
	Liver	50 g	
	Other materials	100 g	

result. The practitioner should remember to combine information from the history and clinical signs before relying on an individual test result to establish a definitive diagnosis.

A toll-free telephone number for toxicology assistance is 1-800-242-3171.

Poison or Analysis Requested	Specimen Required	Amount of Specimen Desired	Comments
Nitrates	Water	50 ml	
	Forage, silage	100 g	
	Whole blood (methemoglobin)	10 ml	
	Other materials	100 g	
	Whole eyeball or aqueous humor	1 ml	
Organophosphorous insecticides	Brain	50 g (cerebrum)	
	Body fat	50 g	
	Stomach contents (composite)	50 g	
	Blood (heparinized)	10 ml	
	Urine	50 ml	
	Feed	100 g	
Oxalates	Fresh forage	6-8 plants	Do *not* chop plants; freeze promptly.
	Kidney (in formalin)	Whole organ	One kidney, both in small animals (qualitative test only)
Phenols	Stomach contents	500 g	Pack in air-tight container.
	Other materials	200 g	
Phenothiazines	Feed or other materials	50 g	
Phosphates	Serum	5 ml	
	Bone	25 g	
	Other materials	100 g	
Thallium	Urine	10 ml	
	Kidney	50 g	
	Liver	50 g	
Urea	Feed	100 g	
	Other materials	500 g	
	See also Ammonia		
Warfarin and other anticoagulants	Whole blood	10 ml	
	Liver	100 g	
	Feed	100 g	
	Other materials	100 g	
Zinc	Liver	50 g	
	Kidney	50 g	
	Other materials	100 g	

*Reprinted with permission from *Current Veterinary Therapy VII* (R.W. Kirk, DVM, Ed.), W.B. Saunders, Philadelphia, PA, 1980.
**A total of 5 ml of nonhemolyzed serum is sufficient to conduct several clinical tests.

CHAPTER 38

Veterinary clinical parasitology

INCREASINGLY, veterinarians are presented with cases requiring treatment, management, and control of parasitisms. This is because the number of companion animals per household in the United States has risen.[1] In addition, a better-educated public is demanding more veterinary services, partially because of greater awareness of the potential for cross-infection between pets and man.

Diagnosis of parasitic infection is most often made by identifying eggs, larvae, cysts, or segments of parasites in feces, blood, or sputum from infected animals. However, clinical experience and research indicate that many factors can influence the outcome of tests for parasites in these stages. An animal may be heavily parasitized, without any parasitic forms being readily detectable. Examples include occult dirofilariasis or massive and even fatal infections of immature and nonfertile roundworms or hookworms in suckling puppies or kittens (clinical disease before the prepatent period).

Gastrointestinal parasites are the most prevalent internal parasites among companion animals. Infection by these parasites is usually diagnosed by means of simple direct fecal smears and concentration techniques such as fecal flotation or sedimentation. Regardless of the technique used, examination of a fresh sample of feces ensures a more accurate diagnosis. As a sample ages, the parasite ova hatch and the larvae deteriorate. In addition, fly larvae and nematodes from the soil invade the sample, thus complicating the diagnosis.

When a fecal sample contains parasitic forms that cannot be identified in the clinic, it should be preserved and submitted to a parasitologist. Fecal samples can be preserved by adding to them 10% formalin or MIF® Solution (Marion Scientific Laboratories). This solution has given more satisfactory results than has formalin. It combines the killing and preserving properties of methiolate, iodine, and formalin with those of glycerin, alcohol, and eosin to form a mixture that kills, fixes, stains, and preserves trophozoites, cysts, and parasite ova.[2]

Direct smears

The most common procedure for diagnosing parasitic infections is concentration of the ova by means of flotation. However, direct smears should also be examined, especially if the feces are soft or liquid. Such samples often contain protozoa that are destroyed beyond recognition by the hypertonic fecal solutions used in concentration techniques. Direct smears also permit detection of ova that are too dense to float, *e.g.* fluke ova.

The direct-smear technique is simple. A small amount of fresh feces is mixed with a few drops of saline solution on a microscope slide, and a coverslip is applied. If staining for protozoa is preferred, a drop of 2% Lugol iodine may be added. The direct smear should be used in conjunction with a concentration technique; it should not routinely be used alone for diagnosis of internal parasitisms.

Concentration techniques

Flotation techniques require mixing of a dense flotation solution with the fecal sample. The parasite ova float to the top of the mixture because they are less dense than the solution. Fecal debris, which is more dense than the solution, sinks to the bottom. Many solutions for fecal flotation are available, including solutions saturated with sucrose, sodium chloride, magnesium sulfate, or zinc sulfate. Procedures for preparing common solutions are listed in Table 1. Commercially prepared solutions are also available. These save time but are more expensive than preparing your own solutions.

A simple fecal flotation is done by thoroughly mixing a small amount of feces with 10 to 25 cc of a saturated fecal flotation solution. (If desired, this mixture can be strained through gauze or cheesecloth.) Next, a straight-sided container, such as a dispensing vial or test tube, is filled with the mixture until a convex meniscus is visible. A glass coverslip or microscope slide is placed on the meniscus and left undisturbed for 5 to 10 minutes. If a glass coverslip is used, it is removed after the waiting period and immediately placed on a microscope slide and examined for ova. If a slide is used, it must be lifted off the meniscus and gently but swiftly inverted. A coverslip is applied, and the slide is examined microscopically.

If desired, a centrifugal flotation method can be used. The feces and flotation solution are mixed in a test tube and centrifuged for two to three minutes. A drop of surface solution is placed on a microscope slide, a coverslip is applied, and the slide is examined microscopically.

Sedimentation concentration techniques are used when the presence of trematode (fluke) parasites is suspected. Because fluke ova are heavier than other helminth ova, they are difficult to recover using flotation techniques. The simple sedimentation procedure is done by mixing a small amount of feces with saline solution and pouring the mixture into a test tube. Next, the mixture is centrifuged for three to five minutes and the supernatant is decanted. A small part of the sediment is collected with a pipette and placed on a microscope slide. A coverslip is applied, and the slide is examined.

The ether-formalin sedimentation technique is outlined in Table 2. Although it is a little more complicated than the simple sedimentation techniques, it is more likely to reveal fluke ova.[3]

Gastrointestinal parasites

Gastrointestinal parasites that most often infect companion animals are shown in Figures 1 through 8. Diarrhea is the most common sign of parasitisms of the gastrointestinal tract. However, intestinal bacteria may contribute to diarrhea in an endoparasitized animal. Thus, treatment with antibiotics alone may cause temporary remission of diarrhea, though the parasites are not affected.

Physaloptera species

Physaloptera canis (dogs), *P. rara* (dogs and cats), and *P. praeputialis* (cats) parasitize primarily the stomach, sometimes causing intermittent vomiting. These endoparasites attach to the mucosa and may cause erosive lesions and catarrhal gastritis. Usually, a parasitized animal has only 1 to 5 parasites. The infection rate in companion animals is low, except in the Midwest where 25 to 30% of the stray dogs were found to be positive.[4,5]

Because few worms are present, very few eggs are shed in the feces. Thus, results of fecal examinations are often negative. The best method for diagnosing this parasitism is by fiberoptic gastroscopy and direct assessment of worm burden. Eggs in the feces resemble hookworm eggs but are smaller and have a thicker shell.

Dichlorvos (Task® —Squibb) is probably the most effective means of treating for *Physaloptera* infection. However, there are no studies to support this hypothesis. Companion animals become infected by ingesting beetles and other winged insects that serve as intermittent hosts.

Ascariasis (roundworms)

Toxocara canis, *T. cati*, and *Toxascaris leonina* are the most widely distributed of the nematodes that parasitize pets. Infection can be transmitted via transplacental, transmammary, and direct oral routes. Migration of the larvae through the lungs may cause verminous pneumonia. Heavy infections can be fatal to puppies, even before the parasites reach adult stages and are able to pass eggs to the stool. Occasionally, large numbers of ascarids cause intestinal obstruction and intussusception.

Toxocara canis, the most common ascarid, is transmitted across the placenta to the fetus during the 34th to 42nd day of pregnancy. It is also transmitted by oral ingestion of larvae from the bitch's milk or from the soil. In female dogs older than 6 months, most of the larvae become encysted in somatic tissue, remaining there until migration is induced by pregnancy.

In addition, *T. canis* can cause visceral larva migrans in man. Infection results from ingestion of eggs containing infective second-stage larvae. Because children are more likely to ingest eggs from the soil, they are at a greater risk of contracting the disease than are adults. Most cases involve children aged 26 to 32 months. Disposing daily of dog feces and excluding dogs from areas where children play reduce the likelihood of infection.

Because of the public health significance of visceral larva migrans and the high incidence of roundworm infection in dogs, all puppies should be treated for roundworms when they are vaccinated. Puppies should be dewormed even if results of fecal tests are negative. Roundworms produce eggs periodically instead of continually. Thus, false negatives are common. The prepatent period, which lasts from the time of infection to demonstration of ova in feces, is usually four to six weeks.

Figure 1 shows roundworm ova as seen on fecal flotation. Treatment can be achieved using any of several safe, commercial anthelmintics.

Ancylostomiasis — uncinariasis (hookworms)

Hookworm infection of dogs is caused by one of three nematodes: *Ancylostoma caninum*, *A. braziliense*, and *Uncinaria stenocephala*. However, only *A. caninum* is hematophagous, and the cardinal sign that differentiates it from the other hookworm infections is anemia. In cats, *A. tubaeformis* is the most common hookworm.

All hookworms of companion animals have a direct life cycle. The parasites are usually transmitted in the dam's milk, though *in utero* transmission can occur. Infection can result from ingestion of infective larvae from the soil or penetration of the skin by infective larvae. The prepatent period is about two weeks. *Ancylostoma braziliense* is the primary cause of cutaneous larva migrans in man, but this disease is relatively insignificant, com-

---

Figure 1—Large, round ova of the roundworm, *Toxocara canis* and smaller oblong ova of the hookworm, *Ancylostoma caninum* (X10 objective magnification).*

Figure 2—Numerous oblong ova of *Ancylostoma caninum* and several darker whipworm ova (*Trichuris vulpis*) with typical bipolar plugs (X10 objective mag.).

Figure 3—Numerous small round coccidia oocysts and one *Ancylostoma caninum* ova (X25 objective mag.).

Figure 4—*Dipylidium caninum* (tapeworm) egg packet (X40 objective magnification).

Figure 5—*Taenia pisiformis* (tapeworm) ova. Note the typical heavy, dark wall (X40 objective mag.).

Figure 6—*Alaria* sp fluke ova from feces of a cat.

Figure 7—*Trichomonas* (protozoan) from a direct saline smear (X100 objective magnification).

Figure 8—*Giardia canis* (protozoan) cysts from direct saline smear (X100 objective magnification).

*Figures 1—5 courtesy of Dr. E. L. Roberson, Dept. of Parasitology, College of Veterinary Medicine, University of Georgia, Athens.

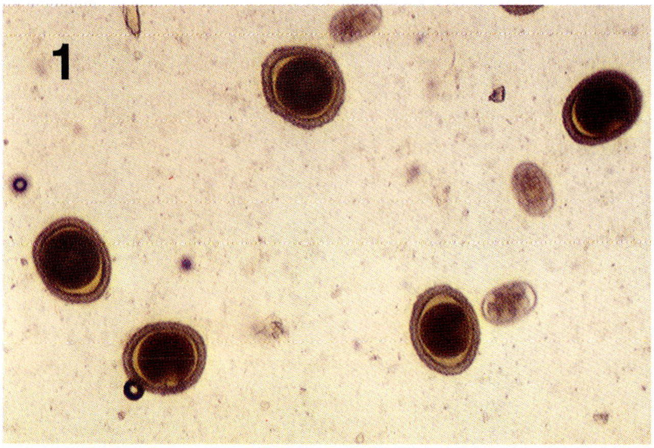
1

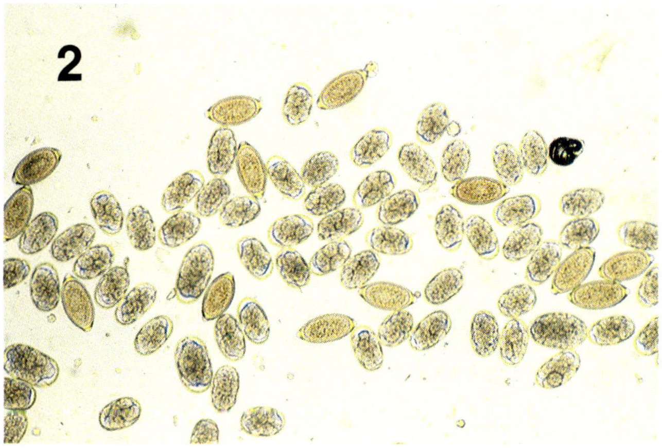
2

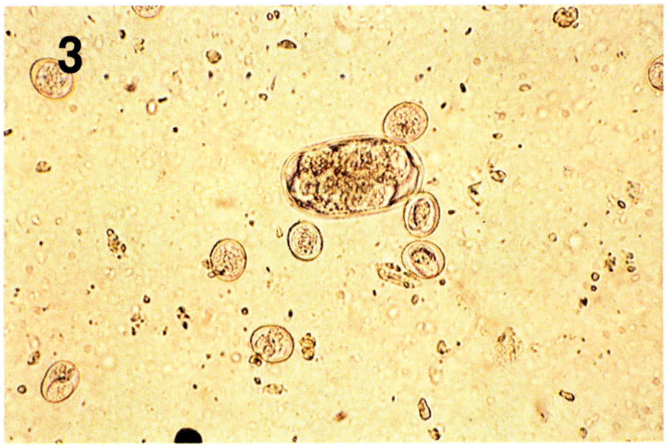
3

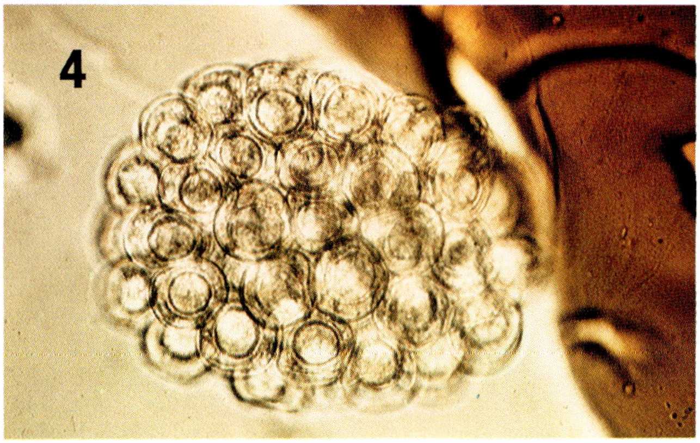
4

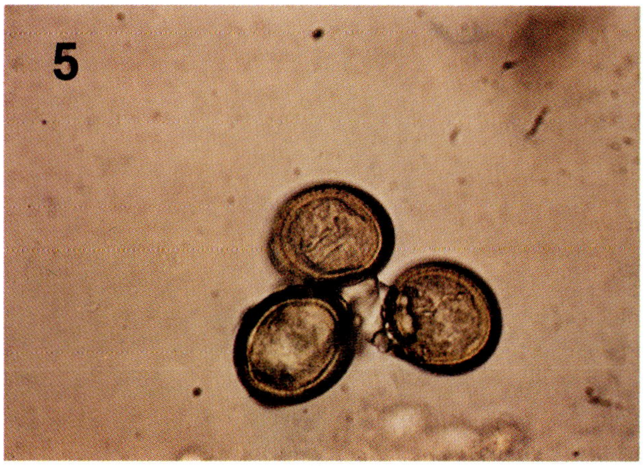
5

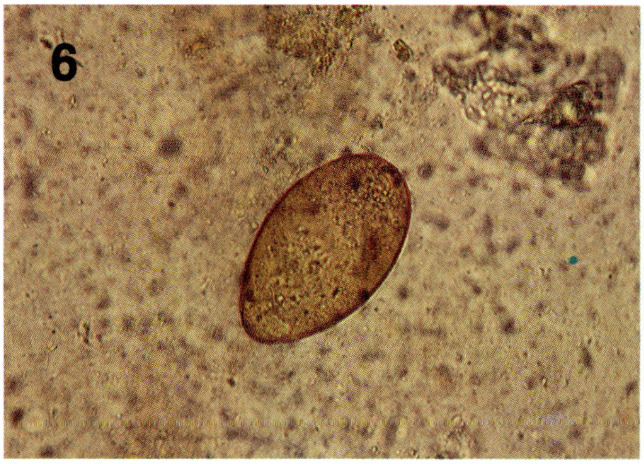
6

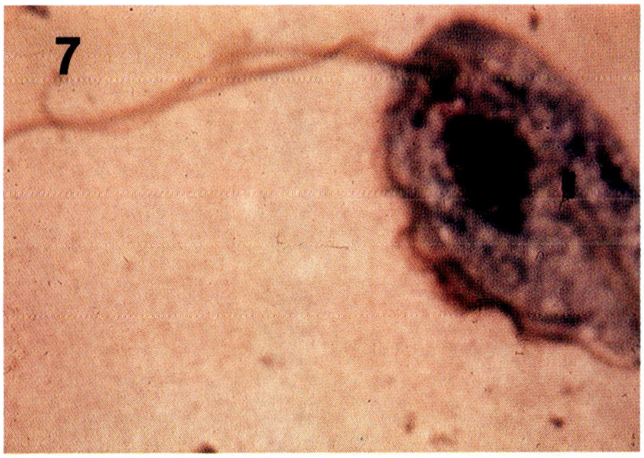
7

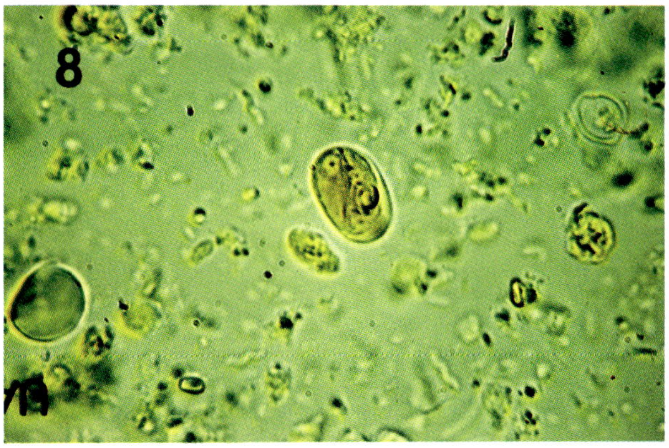
8

pared to visceral larva migrans caused by *T. canis*.

Dichlorvos (31.5 mg/kg) or disophenol (2.2 mg/kg) is used in treatment for hookworm infections in dogs and cats. Blood transfusions may be necessary if the patient is severely anemic. In such cases, the initial aim is to restore blood, fluid, and electrolyte balances and correct any concomitant hypothermia. Only then is the patient given an oral anthelmintic such as dichlorvos, which kills the parasites faster than does disophenol. Hookworm ova are shown in Figures 1 through 3.

Trichuriasis (whipworms)

Trichuris vulpis is the only whipworm found in dogs. It has a direct life cycle. Infection results from ingestion of eggs containing infective larvae. The prepatent period is about four months. The parasite is hematophagous, and has a predilection for the cecum and colon. The whipworm that infects cats is *T. campanula*. It has been reported to occur in cats in South America, Cuba, and the Bahamas.

Because whipworm eggs (*Figure 2*) are resistant to extremes in the environment, the larvae may remain viable in the soil for years. The treatment for whipworm infection is mebendazole (Telmintic™—Pitman-Moore) given at a dosage of 20 mg/kg daily for 7 to 20 days or dichlorvos at a dose of 31.5 mg/kg. Because dichlorvos is contraindicated in dogs with dirofilariasis and because of the high incidence of occult dirofilariasis in parts of the United States, Telmintic is probably preferable. Glycobiarsol (Milibis® -V—Winthrop) at a dosage of 220 mg/kg/day for five days is also effective.

TABLE 1—Solutions for Fecal Flotation

Modified Sheather's Sugar Flotation Solution (Specific Gravity: 1.2 to 1.3)	
Granulated sugar (sucrose)	454 g (1 lb)
Tap Water	355 ml (12 fl oz)
40% Formaldehyde, USP	6 ml
Dissolve sucrose in water over indirect heat. Add formaldehyde to deter growth of molds and yeasts.	
Sodium Chloride (Specific Gravity: 1.2)	
NaCl	36 g
NaCl is dissolved in and brought up to 100 ml with water.	
35% Magnesium Sulfate (Specific Gravity: 1.28)	
$MgSO_4$	35 g
$MgSO_4$ is dissolved in and brought up to 100 ml with water.	
33% Zinc Sulfate (Specific Gravity: 1.18)	
$ZnSO_4$ (anhydrous)	33 g
$ZnSO_4$ is dissolved in and brought up to 100 ml with water.	

Strongyloidiasis

Strongyloides stercoralis can infect both companion animals and man. These nematodes have a predilection for the small intestine and burrow into the intestinal crypts. Adult females produce eggs by parthenogenesis (without fertilization by males). The eggs hatch into larvae within the intestine, and the live larvae are expelled in the feces.

Pets become infected when they ingest larvae or when larvae penetrate the skin. Diagnosis is by finding live *S. stercoralis* larvae in the feces. A Baermann apparatus can be used to concentrate the larvae. Treatment is with Telmintic at a dosage of 20 mg/kg once daily for 7 to 20 days.

Cestodiasis (tapeworms)

Many genera and species of tapeworms infect companion animals in the United States. The prevalence of common types depends on the intermediate host and the environment in which the parasite is found. In most of the United States, the tapeworms transmitted by fleas are most common. However, in some rural areas, tapeworms transmitted by rabbits and rodents are more common.

Dipylidium caninum (Figure 4) is transmitted by fleas and can cause flatulence, diarrhea, and anal pruritus characterized by scooting. Several species of *Taenia* are transmitted to dogs via infected rabbits and rodents. *Taenia* ova from canine

TABLE 2—Method for Ether-Formalin Sedimentation Technique

1. Mix feces in water or saline solution. Using gauze or wire strainer, strain the mixture and collect 10 ml of the emulsion.
2. Centrifuge this material for one minute.
3. Decant and add fresh water or saline solution. Repeat Step 2.
4. Decant and add 10 ml of 10% formalin. Let the mixture stand for 10 minutes.
5. Add 3 ml of ether, apply the stopper, and shake the container vigorously. Centrifuge this mixture for two minutes. Four layers should result: ether on top, a plug of debris, formalin, and sediment.
6. Free the plug of debris with a cotton-tipped applicator and decant.
7. Collect the sediment and examine it microscopically for fluke ova.

feces are shown in Figure 5.

Diphyllobothrium latum is transmitted to dogs and man by infected fish in northern states. *Echinococcus granulosus* is a cestode of public health significance that can cause formation of large cysts in animals and man.

Either the oral or injectable form of Droncit® (Haver-Lockhart) is effective treatment for tapeworm infections. Scoloban® (Wellcome) given orally at a dosage of 25 to 50 mg/kg is also effective.

Trematodiasis

Alaria species of flukes affect the intestines of dogs and cats (*Figure 6*). The flukes attach to the intestine and can cause catarrhal enteritis. Cats can be infected with other species of liver flukes, including *Amphimerus felineus* and *Platynosomum* species. The clinical significance of these species is questionable because fluke ova are found in many asymptomatic cats in southern United States. Occasionally, however, these species can cause significant hepatobiliary disease. No effective drugs exist for treatment of fluke infections in companion animals. However, some positive results have been achieved by administering albendazole or fenbendazole at a dosage of 32 mg/kg/day for seven days, then repeating the regimen after three weeks.

Nanophyetus salmincola can infest the intestines of dogs in northwestern states where salmonoid fish can harbor the infective larval forms. The flukes themselves cause few problems, but they can carry rickettsial pathogens such as *Neorickettsia helminthoeca* and the agent of Elokomin fluke fever, which can cause fatal enteritis in dogs. Historically, the disease has been called *salmon poisoning*. Treatment is with tetracyclines and is aimed at destroying the rickettsia, rather than the trematodes.

Paragonimus kellicotti is a lung fluke that can infect many species of animals. This parasite, found primarily in the Midwest, can produce pulmonary bullae and lead to fatal pneumothorax.

Flagellates

Flagellated protozoa of companion animals, principally *Giardia canis*, *G. cati*, and *Trichomonas* sp (*Figure 7*), multiply in the intestinal tract. The vegetative multiplying forms of *Giardia* (trophozoites) can occur in the lumen of the small intestine and attach to mucosal cells. While passing through the large bowel, the parasites encyst. The cyst stage, as well as the trophozoite stages, may be detected in the feces (*Figure 8*).

Because the hypertonic solutions used for fecal flotation cause flagellated protozoan parasites to crenate beyond recognition, they are diagnosed from direct saline smears. Treatment is with metronidazole at 70 mg/kg/day for five days.

Coccidiosis

The coccidia that most often infect dogs and cats are *Isospora canis*, *I. felis*, *I. rivolta*, and *Eimeria* species. The tiny oocysts of *Toxoplasma gondii* are found only in cats and are indistinguishable from other related species of *Isospora*.[6] Diagnosis of coccidiosis is based on demonstration of the characteristic oocysts (*Figure 3*) in feces of infected animals. The oocysts may occur sporadically in asymptomatic animals, which can serve as carriers. Pronounced disease processes resulting from overwhelming numbers of coccidial organisms are seen primarily in young puppies and kittens.

Treatment is with sulfonamides such as sulfadimethoxine (Albon® —Hoffmann-LaRoche). A loading dose of 55 mg/kg is followed by a dosage of 27.5 mg/kg/day for 10 to 14 days. Tetracyclines are effective when given at a dosage of 16 mg/kg three times daily. However, the tetracycline drugs can be incorporated into the enamel of the deciduous teeth and the forming permanent teeth, thus causing discoloration of the permanent dentition.

Comment

Diagnosis of Gastrointestinal Parasitism in Dogs and Cats, published by Ralston Purina, is an excellent source of photomicrographs of all the ova, cyst, and larval forms of gastrointestinal parasites of small animals.[6]

REFERENCES

1. Nowell, I.: *The Dog Crisis.* St. Martin's Press, New York, N.Y., 1978.
2. Price, D.L.: Comparison of Three Collection-Preservation Methods for Detection of Intestinal Parasites. *J. Clin. Microbiol.*, Dec. 1981; pp 656-660.
3. Richie, L.S. *et al*: A Comparison of the Zinc Sulfate and MGL (Formalin-Ether) Techniques. *J. Parasitol. 38*:16-17; 1952.
4. Ehrenford, F.A.: Diagnosis of *Physaloptera* in Dogs by Stool Examination. *J. Parasitol. 40* (suppl):16; 1954.
5. Levine, N.D.: *Nematode Parasites of Domestic Animals and of Man*, 2nd Ed. Burgess Publishing, Minneapolis, Minn., 1973.
6. Williams, J.F.; Zajac, A.: *Diagnosis of Gastrointestinal Parasitism in Dogs and Cats*, Ralston-Purina Co., St. Louis, Mo., 1980.

CHAPTER 39

Biopsy techniques

Biopsy is the removal of tissue or other material from the living body for examination by means of histologic, cytologic, or microbiologic techniques. Biopsy is an indispensable method of clinical evaluation. Often it is the principal means of diagnosing diseases, particularly those that can only be identified on the basis of specific morphologic alterations (*e.g.* hepatic cirrhosis, eosinophilic myositis).

In the usual clinical setting, history, physical examination, radiography, and biochemical laboratory procedures are used to identify: 1) the disease process or 2) the specific site of disease. Many disease syndromes then can be identified further by biopsy of the affected organ. In many cases when the specific diagnosis is known, biopsy aids in determining whether the disease process is reversible or progressively irreversible. If the condition is reversible, biopsy can be used to ascertain whether partial or complete recovery can be expected.

The patient should be evaluated carefully before biopsy to ensure that information gained by the procedure will outweigh any potential risk to the patient. Because most clinicians are experienced in performing biopsies and biopsy instrumentation has been improved substantially, the proven value of the procedure generally outweighs any risk to the patient. Potential contraindications to biopsy include hemostasis disorders, damaged biopsy instruments, the clinician's inexperience, and malignant neoplasms.

Hemorrhage is one of the most serious complications that can follow a biopsy. Any abnormalities in the patient's hemostasis should be corrected before internal biopsies are performed. Any hemorrhagic disorder that cannot be corrected precludes biopsy of internal organs, except for bone marrow. Procedures for determining hemostasis and coagu-

Figure 1—The Franklin modified Vim Silverman needle.

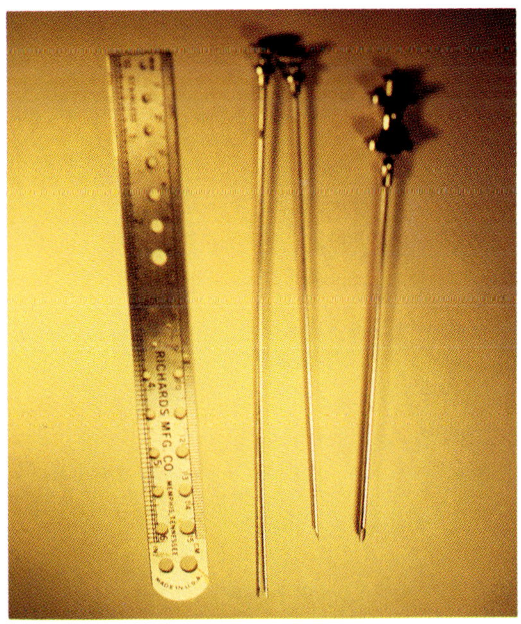

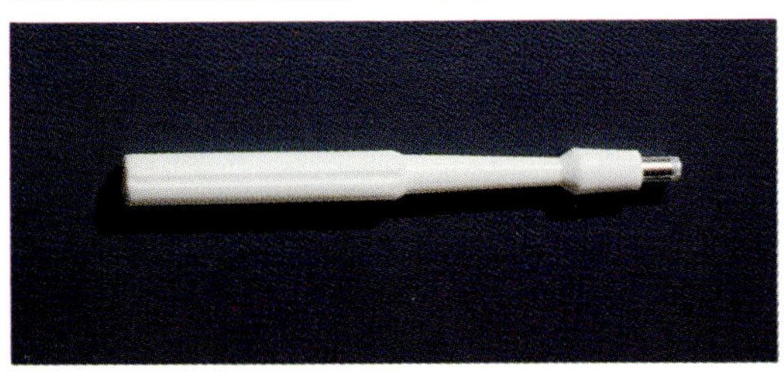

Figure 2—The Baker biopsy punch.

lation defects have been discussed elsewhere.[1]

Inexperienced clinicians and faulty equipment also constitute potential problems. Practitioners who are inexperienced at performing biopsies on internal organs should practice the procedures on cadavers. Damaged needles or biopsy forceps may: 1) make it impossible to obtain an adequate sample or 2) result in repeated, futile, dangerous attempts to obtain a specimen.

Biopsy of neoplasms that are probably malignant may result in dissemination of cancer cells along the biopsy tract during withdrawal of the needle and in destruction of the neoplasm capsule. Results of experimental studies and clinical observations indicate that this is more a theoretical than actual complication.[2] However, hemangiosarcoma of the spleen may be a notable exception.[3]

Methods of biopsy

Biopsies may be classified as excisional, incisional, aspiration, or needle punch.

Excisional biopsy

Excisional biopsy is the complete surgical excision of the affected lesion or tissue. This is the preferred method of biopsy, if it does not interfere with normal function of the target tissue or organ system, or if proper function of the tissue is not necessary. Excisional biopsies are indicated for use in 1) accessible solitary lesions in most organ systems and 2) solitary or multiple lesions in organs or tissues not necessary for maintenance of life, *e.g.* spleen, testes, ovaries, uterus. A major advantage of this procedure is that it incorporates both diagnosis and treatment.

Incisional biopsy

This biopsy procedure is the surgical removal of a *portion* of a lesion, tissue, or organ system. Incisional biopsies are preferred when the lesion is too large to excise or when the lesion diffusely involves a vital organ system. This procedure yields more tissue than does an aspiration biopsy. Also, the normal architecture of the specimen is maintained for histologic evaluation.

Aspiration biopsy

This method involves the use of a syringe to apply negative pressure to remove from the body cells or bits of tissue and/or fluid through a needle or catheter. By strict definition, aspiration biopsy includes taking blood samples by venipuncture and urine samples by catheterization or cystocentesis. However, the term is generally used to refer to the aspiration of cells from tumor masses, lymph nodes, and body cavities.

Aspiration biopsy is simple and quick to perform and is safe for the patient. Often the results are sufficient for a specific diagnosis (*e.g.* lymphosarcoma, melanoma, mast cell tumor) or for differentiation of inflammation and neoplasia. The primary disadvantage of aspiration biopsy, as compared to incisional or excisional biopsies, is that the architecture of the specimen is altered; only detached cells and fluid are available for study.

Needle-punch biopsy

Needle-punch biopsy is the removal of a core of tissue using the cutting action of a biopsy needle. This method permits collection of several samples from different areas and several depths. In addition, the normal architecture of the tissue specimen is preserved, thus facilitating histologic study. A needle-punch biopsy is generally safer than an incisional or excisional biopsy and yields more useful information than does aspiration biopsy. The tissue specimen obtained is usually large enough to permit preparation of gentle impression smears and cultures for cytologic and microbiologic study. The techniques for impression smears and exfoliative cytology have been discussed.[4]

Many instruments are available for performing needle-punch biopsies. We prefer the Franklin modified Vim Silverman biopsy needle (V. Mueller Co., Chicago, Ill.) (*Figure 1*) or the disposable Vim

Tru-Cut biopsy needle (Baxter Laboratories, Morton Grove, Ill.) The Franklin needle is made of stainless steel. It consists of an outer 14-gauge needle cannula, a detachable stylet, and cutting prongs (*Figure 1*). The Vim Tru-Cut consists of a 14-gauge needle with plastic handles and a rod for cutting internal specimens. The movable parts of this needle are incorporated into a one-piece interlocking assembly that requires less practice and dexterity to use than the separate components of the Franklin needle.

The general technique for using either needle is essentially the same. The skin over the target organ or tissue should be clipped, cleaned as for aseptic surgery, and infiltrated with a local anesthetic. General anesthesia may be preferred, depending on the patient's temperament and accessibility of the lesion.

A stab incision just large enough to accommo date the biopsy needle is made in the skin, and the needle is advanced until it touches the target organ. Next, the stylet is removed (in the case of the Franklin needle), and the cutting prongs are inserted through the needle. The needle should be positioned so that the exact route of the prongs is known, care being taken to avoid damage to vital structures. The cutting prongs are thrust into the tissue, making a clean, swift cut. The cannula is advanced to cover the cutting prongs, and the entire needle is removed. If the Vim Tru-cut needle is used, the tip of the built-in cutting rod serves as the stylet. Thus, the steps of removing the stylet and inserting the cutting prongs are eliminated.

Common sites of biopsy

Liver

Biopsy of the liver is best performed using the *key-hole* method. This involves placement of a stab incision on the ventral midline behind the xiphoid cartilage. The incision should be just large enough to permit entry of the index finger, which is used to palpate the lobes of the liver, the gallbladder, stomach, and kidney for abnormalities. Another stab incision, for insertion of the biopsy needle, is made 2 to 3 inches to the left of the midline. The left lateral hepatic lobe is compressed against the lateral abdominal wall, and the needle is advanced until it touches the surface of the lobe. The procedure then is continued as previously described.

The left lateral hepatic lobe is preferred because it is the largest lobe of the liver and because the gallbladder is on the opposite side, thus reducing the chance of it being punctured. If a solitary lesion is palpated by the index finger, the lesion itself should be the target of the biopsy.

Kidney

The technique for obtaining a biopsy specimen of the kidney is the same as for obtaining a liver specimen except that the animal is placed in lateral recumbency and the key hole incision for the index finger is made over the caudal pole of the kidney. In cats, a blind percutaneous technique can often be used because both the right and left kidneys can be identified and immobilized by digital palpation of the abdomen.

Lymph node

Biopsy of lymph nodes is best done by means of total surgical excision or needle aspiration. Needle aspiration and cytologic examination have been described.[4]

Skin biopsy

Biopsy of skin lesions can safely be made by excisional, incisional, or needle-punch techniques. In generalized dermatologic conditions, the punch biopsy is preferred. Several instruments are available for performing skin-punch biopsies. We prefer the Baker biopsy punch (Chester A. Baker Laboratories, Miami, Fla.) (*Figure 2*). With its circular cutting edge and plastic handle, the instrument resembles a cookie cutter. It is available in various diameters, but in our experience, the 3.5-or 4.0-mm sizes are most useful. The instrument is drilled by rotary movement into the skin. When all layers of the skin have been penetrated, the instrument is withdrawn, and the specimen is gently lifted. Scissors are used to cut the specimen away from the subcutis. Generally, this procedure can be accomplished easily using only local anesthesia. One nonabsorbable suture is used to close the wound.

Bone marrow

The techniques and cytology of bone marrow biopsies have been discussed elsewhere.[5]

Comments

Biopsy specimens can be fixed in 10% buffered formalin for routine histology. If immunofluorescent studies are planned, the specimens should be fixed in Michel's fixative. For electron-microscopic studies, the fixative of choice is 3% glutaraldehyde.

An excellent reference for a more detailed explanation of biopsy techniques is *Veterinary Clinics of North America* (May 1974).

REFERENCES

1. Goldston, R.T. *et al*: Hemostasis/Coagulation: A Clinical Approach to Bleeding Disorders. *VM/SAC* 77(8):1165-1170; 1982.
2. Engzell, U. *et al*: Investigation on Tumor Spread in Connection with Aspiration Biopsy. *Acta. Radiol.* *10*:385-398; 1971.
3. Osborne, C.A. (ed.): *Veterinary Clinics of North America*, Vol. 2, No. 4. W.B. Saunders, Philadelphia, Pa.; 1974.
4. Seybold, I.M. *et al*: Exfoliative Cytology. *VM/SAC* 77(7):1029-1033; 1982.
5. Seybold, I.M. *et al*: Examination of the Bone Marrow. *VM/SAC* 75(10):1517-1521; 1980.

CHAPTER 40

Hemostasis/coagulation:

a clinical approach to bleeding disorders

A NUMBER of specific heritable and acquired bleeding disorders affect companion animals. These hemorrhagic disorders as seen in man are well documented. In recent years, their occurrence in companion animals has attracted considerable interest and attention.[1-3] Proper understanding of hemorrhagic disorders necessitates a basic knowledge of normal hemostasis and coagulation.

Normal hemostasis/coagulation mechanisms

Companion animals are often subjected to traumatic episodes that cause hemorrhage. However, due to the presence of an efficient hemostasis/coagulation mechanism, severe blood loss seldom results from such episodes.

This complex hemostasis/coagulation mechanism involves the interaction between blood vessel contractility, platelet (thrombocyte) function, and plasma clotting factors. The immediate reaction to injury of a blood vessel is vasoconstriction; this reduces both the total blood flow through the damaged vessel and the total damaged surface area that must be "plugged" by the coagulation mechanism. The platelets form an emergency plug by occluding the defect, and the plasma clotting factors undergo a cascade of reactions that lead to formation of a fibrin clot. The fibrin clot strengthens the platelet plug and serves as a framework for the process of fibroblastic repair. The procedure for determining the activated clotting time (ACT) as outlined in Table 1 is a whole-blood clotting test; it is good for screening for bleeding tendencies. The normal ACT for dogs is 60 to 100 seconds. If the ACT is abnormal, other, specific tests are indicated.

Platelet function and laboratory evaluation

When normal platelets contact extravascular collagen, platelet aggregator substances are released that cause more platelets to aggregate and adhere to the damaged vascular walls. This process continues until the defect in the vessel is closed by a primary platelet plug. Platelets also release *platelet factor 3* which accelerates the function of the plasma clotting factors. After the clot is formed, the platelets release the protein *thrombasthenin*, which aids in normal clot retraction.

Hemorrhagic syndromes resulting from platelet disorders are characterized by superficial bleeding such as epistaxis, gingival hemorrhage, hemarthrosis, and petechial and ecchymotic hemorrhages of the skin. These syndromes in companion animals can be divided into 1) *thrombocytopenias*, associated with reduced numbers of platelets, and 2) *thrombocytopathies*, characterized by normal platelet counts but abnormal platelet function.

Thrombocytopenias

Thrombocytopenia is the most common cause of hemorrhagic diathesis in companion animals; it is seen when platelet counts drop below 50,000/

μl. Examination of a stained blood smear can reveal suspect thrombocytopenia as the platelet number should be approximately 1 per 20 to 30 erythrocytes. Thrombocytopenia can be easily confirmed by a platelet count performed with a hemacytometer and a precalibrated dilution system (Unopette® —Becton-Dickinson), using the same procedure as used for the white blood cell count.[4] The normal platelet count for companion animals is 150,000 to 400,000 μl.

Thrombocytopenia can be caused by several different mechanisms. *Hypoproliferative thrombocytopenias* result from reduced production of platelets by the bone marrow. They can occur in association with the administration of drugs such as estrogens, with infiltrating neoplastic diseases such as lymphoreticular neoplasias, and with transient viremias including live-virus vaccines. *Destruction thrombocytopenias* are caused by shortened lifespan of platelets. They can result from such immune-mediated disorders as immune-mediated thrombocytopenia (idiopathic thrombocytopenia purpura) and systemic lupus erythematosus. Other causes of destruction thrombocytopenia are over-consumption of platelets as occurs in disseminated intravascular coagulation and acute massive hemorrhage.

TABLE 1—How to Measure Activated Clotting Time

1. Pre-warm two ACT Vacutainer tubes (Becton-Dickinson) to 37 C in a water bath or heater.
2. By clean venipuncture withdraw the first few drops of blood in one Vacutainer tube and discard it.
3. Start timing with a stopwatch when blood enters the second ACT tube.
4. Mix contents of the tube by inverting the tube five times.
5. Replace the tube in the heating block or water bath.
6. After one minute, remove the tube to check for clotting.
7. Replace the tube in the heating block.
8. Recheck the tube every five seconds until a clot is detected.
9. Record the time in seconds.

TABLE 2—Plasma Clotting Factors

International Classification*	Commonly Used Synonyms
Factor I	Fibrinogen
Factor II	Prothrombin
Factor III	Tissue thromboplastin
Factor IV	Calcium
Factor V	Proaccelerin
Factor VII	Proconvertin
Factor VIII	Antihemophilic factor
Factor IX	Christmas factor
Factor X	Stuart factor
Factor XI	Plasma thromboplastin antecedent
Factor XII	Hageman factor
Factor XIII	Fibrin stabilizing factor

*As recommended by the International Committee for the Nomenclature of Blood Clotting Factors (1962). No factor has been assigned to number VI.

Thrombocytopathies

In thrombocytopathies, the function of platelets is impaired but the platelet count is normal. Inherited thrombocytopathies include thrombasthenia (Glanzman disease), a deficiency of platelet factor 3. Its occurrence in Otter Hounds, Basset Hounds, and Scottish Terriers has been described. Acquired thrombocytopathies are seen often and are associated with aspirin ingestion and uremia. Aspirin inactivates enzymes (cycle-oxygenases) required for aggregation of platelets. Uremia prompts the vascular endothelium to produce excess prostacyclin,[5] the most potent known inhibitor of platelets.

Thrombocytopathies should be suspected in bleeding disorders when routine coagulation screening tests and platelet counts are normal. Thrombocytopathy can be confirmed by demostrating prolonged bleeding and clot-retraction time.

The bleeding-time test measures bleeding time from a standard puncture wound of hairless skin or the oral mucosa. A puncture wound is made with a disposable lancet, and a stopwatch is started. Bleeding is allowed to proceed without pressure.

When the bleeding slows, the wound is touched gently with filter paper at 30-second intervals. When blood no longer stains the filter paper, the watch is stopped and the time recorded. The normal range is up to five minutes. For comparison, the test should also be done on a control animal.

The clot-retraction test measures the time required for a whole blood clot to retract from the sides of a test tube and serum to begin collecting on the top. Within 12 to 24 hours, clear serum should be evident above and around the clot in the test tube. Failure of the clot to retract in that time indicates thrombocytopenia or thrombocytopathy.

Treatment of thrombocytopenias and thrombocytopathies depends on the inciting cause. Most thrombocytopathies result from aspirin or similar drug therapy or, secondarily, from uremia. In such cases, administration of the offending drugs is discontinued. In the case of uremia, treatment is given as previously described.[6] Most thrombocytopenias appear to be immune-mediated or to result from a transient viremia. In these cases, the bone marrow should be examined. If megakaryocytes, the precursors of platelets, are present, the platelets are either being immunologically destroyed or sequestered. If megakaryocytes are not present, the stem cell has probably been damaged by virus infection, or bone marrow has been replaced by an infiltrative process such as lymphoreticular neoplasia, amyloidosis, or myelofibrosis. In those cases, the prognosis is poor at best.

Treatment for immune-mediated thrombocytopenias consists of prednisolone at a dosage of 0.5 to 1 mg/lb twice daily. If no response is noted and splenomegaly exists, the spleen should be removed. In refractory cases, other immunosuppressant agents such as cyclophosphamide (Cytoxan® — Mead Johnson) or azathioprine (Imuran® —Burroughs Wellcome) can be given at a dosage of 0.5 to 1 mg/lb/day. If the thrombocytopenia has resulted in severe blood-loss anemia, whole-blood transfusions or platelet-rich plasma transfusions are beneficial. Platelet-rich plasma can easily be obtained

TABLE 3—How to Perform the Test for One-Stage Prothrombin Time (PT)

Reagents

1. Thromboplastin. This reagent is commercially prepared, usually in the form of a suspension of acetone-dried extract of brain tissue.
2. Calcium chloride 0.02 molar. Many preparations are available in which the thromboplastin and calcium are mixed and ready to use.

Procedure

1. Place two test tubes in a warm water bath.
2. Add 0.2 ml of thromboplastin-calcium mixture to each tube, or add 0.1 ml thromboplastin and 0.1 ml calcium chloride.
3. Allow tubes to warm for about 30 seconds.
4. Taking one tube at a time, add 0.1 ml of sample plasma by blowing it quickly into the thromboplastin mixture. Start stopwatch at the same time.
5. Leave the tube in the water bath for 10 seconds while continuously and gently agitating it.
6. Remove the tube. Hold it in front of a bright light and slightly tilt it every second until a clot appears. Then, stop the watch.
7. Test each sample twice and average results.
8. Include a normal plasma control with each batch. Results are reported in seconds. The control time should also be recorded. Normal values for dogs range from 7 to 9 seconds.

TABLE 4—How to Determine Activated Partial Thromboplastin Time (PTT)

1. In duplicate 10 mm x 75 mm test tubes, add 0.1 ml test plasma and 0.1 ml commercial activated cephalin reagent (Ortho, Hyland, Dade, or Warner-Lambert).
2. Place tubes in water bath at 37 C and incubate for 3 to 10 minutes according to instructions for commercial cephalin reagent. Quickly add 0.1 ml M/40 calcium chloride.
3. Start stopwatch immediately as you add calcium chloride.
4. Time clot formation. Normal values for dogs range from 18 to 30 seconds, depending on the source of commercial cephalin reagent. Times vary with the species; be sure to run a homologous control sample with all patient samples.

TABLE 5—How to Determine Thrombin Time (TT)

1. In duplicate 10 mm x 75 mm test tubes, add 0.2 ml test plasma.
2. Place tubes in water bath at 37 C. Quickly add 0.1 ml bovine thrombin — 10 units/ml (Ortho, Hyland, Dade, or Warner-Lambert).
3. Start stopwatch immediately as you add thrombin. Normal values for dogs range from 9 to 12 seconds.

by allowing whole blood in acid citrate dextrose anticoagulant to settle out and then gently withdrawing the supernatant plasma.

Plasma clotting factors and laboratory evaluation

The plasma clotting factors contribute to hemostasis by means of a cascade of chemical reactions that ultimately yields a stabilized fibrin clot. This clot stabilizes the initial "platelet plug" and serves as a matrix for fibroblastic repair of the defect in the vessel. Formation of fibrin can occur by two distinct chemical reaction pathways: 1) *intrinsic* (intravascular) and 2) *extrinsic*.

Figure 1—Intrinsic, Extrinsic and Common Pathway Coagulation Reactions

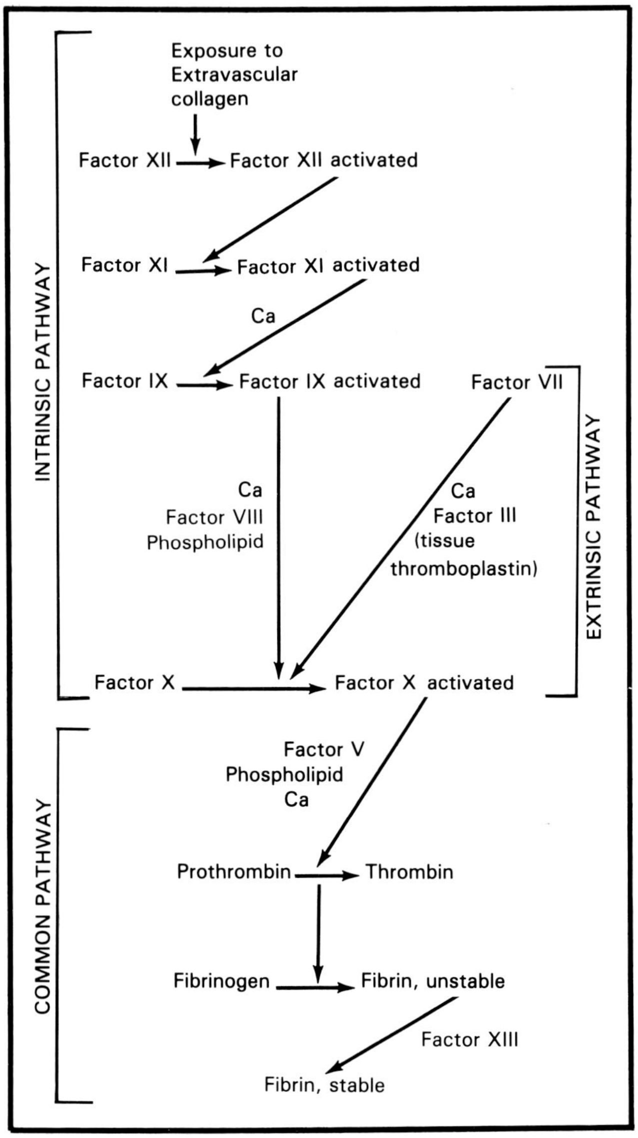

In the intrinsic pathway, all the necessary chemical factors are present in an inactive form in normal plasma. Activation of Hageman factor (Factor XII), by exposure to extravascular collagen, will sequentially allow activation of the other factors until fibrin is formed. In the extrinsic pathway, initiation of the clotting reaction requires release of an extravascular "tissue factor" from injured cells. This is a faster method of fibrin formation that occurs when major tissue damage has been sustained.

Both the intrinsic and extrinsic systems share a common pathway for the final reactions leading to fibrin formation. Because the coagulation reactions of the plasma clotting factors depend on sequential chemical reactions, deficiencies of a single clotting factor can cause hemorrhagic disorders.

Table 2 lists numerically the plasma clotting factors and common synonyms for them. Figure 1 illustrates the enzyme cascades leading to stabilized fibrin formation.

In the intrinsic pathway, Factor XII becomes activated when exposed to extravascular collagen. Activated Factor XII activates Factor XI which, in the presence of calcium, activates Factor IX. A hereditary deficiency of Factor IX causes hemophilia B. Activated Factor IX activates Factor X in the presence of calcium, a phospholipid, and Factor VIII. A hereditary deficiency of Factor VIII presents as the classic hemophilia A.

Factor X can be activated more directly and rapidly in the presence of major tissue damage by the release of tissue thromboplastin. In this, the extrinsic pathway, Factor VII, calcium, and tissue thromboplastin (Factor III) directly interact to form activated Factor X.

When Factor X has been activated, the pathway is the same for the intrinsic and the extrinsic systems and is called the *common* pathway. Activated Factor X converts prothrombin to thrombin which, in turn, converts fibrinogen to unstable fibrin. The unstable fibrin is converted to stable fibrin by Factor XIII.

A hemorrhagic disease can be traced to the intrinsic pathway, extrinsic pathway, or common pathway by means of three laboratory tests: prothrombin time (PT), partial thromboplastin time (PTT), and thrombin time (TT). These tests can be done in any well-equipped in-hospital laboratory, but results usually are more reliable if they are done by a commercial laboratory. Methods for performing the tests are outlined in Tables 3 through 5.

Figure 2—Characteristics and Diagnosis of Hemorrhagic Disorders

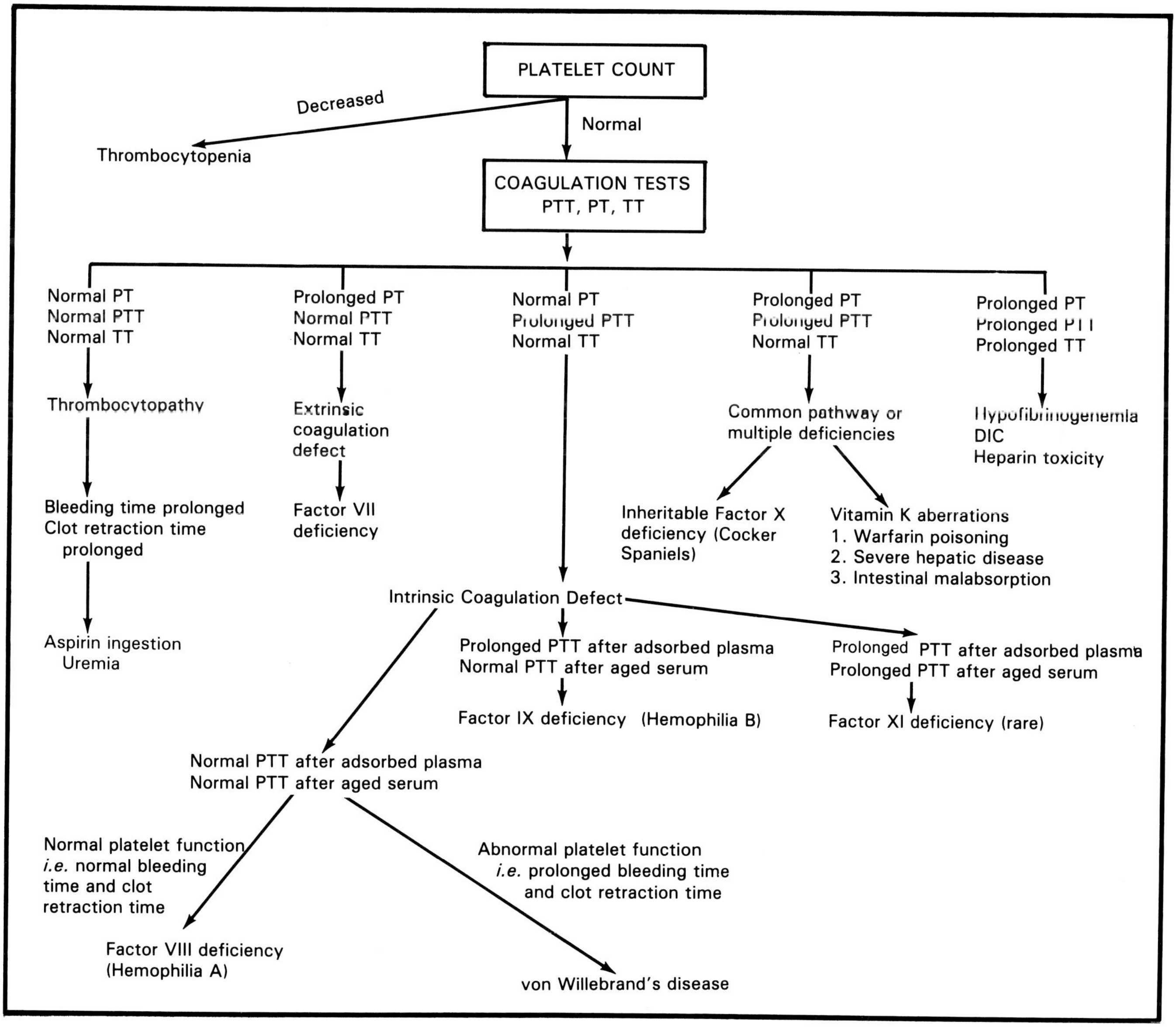

When samples are to be sent to a commercial laboratory, the blood is carefully collected by venipuncture to prevent contamination by tissue fluids. The sample is placed in a tube containing 1 part 3.8% trisodium citrate to 9 parts blood. Plasma should be drawn off and immediately tested or frozen. A control sample should be submitted with the patient's sample. Normal PT for companion animals is 7 to 9 seconds. Normal PTT is 18 to 30 seconds, and normal TT is 9 to 12 seconds.

Intrinsic coagulation defects are characterized by a normal platelet count, PT, and TT, but a prolonged PTT. Three well-described, severely hemorrhagic diseases of dogs fall into this category. They are hemophilia A (Factor VIII deficiency), hemophilia B (Factor IX deficiency) and von Willebrand disease (Factor VIII deficiency and platelet abnormality). To differentiate the hemophilia A and B disorders, the PTT test is repeated after adding normal-aged serum that contains Factor IX but not Factor VIII. The PTT is again repeated after the addition of adsorbed plasma containing Factor VIII but not Factor IX. A normal PTT after aged serum has been added indicates that the hemorrhagic diathesis is hemophilia B. If the PTT is normal only after the addition of adsorbed plasma, hemophilia A is indicated. Specific diagnosis of Factor VIII or IX deficiencies can also be made from results of a specific factor assay.

A Factor XII deficiency in cats[7] has been reported that does not result in clinical hemorrhage. Factor XII is normally absent in marine mammals, birds, and reptiles.

Factor XI deficiency in Springer Spaniels[8] has been reported, but it is rare. A definitive diagnosis depends on specific Factor XI assay, but the deficiency is suspected in cases of hemorrhage in which the only abnormality is a prolonged PTT that is not correctable by either absorbed plasma or aged serum.

Extrinsic coagulation defects are characterized by normal platelet count, PTT, and TT, but a prolonged PT. The only reported cases have been Factor VII deficiencies in Beagles and a single Malamute. Bruising, but not clinical hemorrhage, occurs with this disorder.

Multiple deficiencies and deficiencies in the common pathway are characterized by normal platelet count and TT, but prolonged PT and PTT. The only known heritable common-pathway deficiency in dogs is Factor X deficiency in Cocker Spaniels.[9] Acquired multiple deficiencies, however, are common. They include the hemorrhagic disorders associated with vitamin K deficiency, warfarin toxicity, severe hepatic disease, and severe prolonged intestinal malabsorption disease. Clotting factors that depend on vitamin K are Factors II, VII, IX and X.

With fibrinogen disorders, platelet counts are normal; PT, PTT, and TT are prolonged. The most commonly occurring fibrinogen disorder is hypofibrinogenemia secondary to such consumptive coagulopathies as disseminated intravascular coagulation. The normal fibrinogen level in dogs is 300 mg/dl ± 100 mg/dl; 50 mg/dl or less is considered a significant hypofibrinogenemia. Figure 2 illustrates the differentiation of the common hemorrhagic disorders using the following coagulation screening tests: 1) platelet numbers, 2) prothrombin time, 3) partial thromboplastin time, and 4) thrombin time.

REFERENCES

1. Rebar, A.H.; Boon, G.D.: A Diagnostic Approach to Bleeding Disorders in the Dog. *Proc. 47th Ann. Mtg. AAHA*, 1980; pp 125-129.
2. Dodds, W.J.; Kaneko, J.J.: Hemostasis and Blood Coagulation. In *Clinical Biochemistry of Domestic Animals.* (J.J. Kaneko; C.E. Cornelius, eds). Academic Press, New York, N.Y., 1970.
3. Dodds, W.J.: Bleeding Disorders. In *Textbook of Veterinary Internal Medicine.* (Ettinger, S.J., ed). W.B. Saunders Co., Philadelphia, Pa., 1975.
4. Wilkes, R.D. *et al*: The Basic Clinical Pathology Laboratory-7: Preparation of the Leukocytic Hemogram. *VM/SAC 75*(7):1101-1107; 1980.
5. Remuzzi, G. *et al*: Prostacyclin-like Activity and Bleeding in Renal Failure. *Lancet* 2 (8050):1195-1197; 1976.
6. Goldston, R.T. *et al*: The Clinical Pathology Laboratory -16: Evaluation of Renal Function—3. Evaluation, Treatment, and Management of Patients with Chronic Renal Failure. *VM/SAC 76*(4): 474-477; 1981.
7. Green, R.A.; White, F.: Feline Factor XII (Hageman) Deficiency. *Am. J. Vet. Res.* Vol. 38; No. 6; 1977.
8. Dodds, W.J.; Kull, J.E.: Canine Factor XI (Plasma Thromboplastin Antecedent) Deficiency. *J. Lab. Clin. Med. 78*:746; 1971.
9. Rowsell, H.C. *et al*: A Disorder Resembling Hemophilia B (Christmas Disease) in Dogs. *JAVMA 137*:247; 1960.

GLOSSARY

Absolute Shift—When the number of a specific leukocyte is more or less than normal for the species.

Acanthocyte—A spiculated or spiny erythrocyte.

Achlorhydria—A deficiency in the production of hydrochloric acid by the parietal epitheial cells of the stomach.

Achromatic Objective—A lens of laboratory quality corrected for two colors of chromatic abberation and one color of spherical abberation.

Achromatic Substage Condenser—A condenser for use with achromatic and apochromatic objectives.

Agar—A substance used to support microbial growth.

Agranulocyte—A leukocyte without definite cytoplasmic granules.

Allergen—An antigen that stimulates the formaation of IgE antibodies and trigger the release of the substances from mast cells that cause an allergic reaction.

Amylase—An enzyme produced in its active form by the pancreas that breaks down polysaccharides into monosaccharides and disaccharides.

Amylorrhea—Undigested starch granules in the stool in amounts greater than normal.

Anabolism—Constructive metabolism whereby simple compounds are converted into body fats and proteins.

Anagen—The growth phase of a hair follicle.

Analgesic—A medication used to relieve pain.

Anemia—A decrease of more than two standard deviations below the mean normal in hemoglobin value, the packed cell volume, or the erythrocyte count.

- Aplastic—An anemia induced by impaired erythrocyte production by the bone marrow.
- Hemolytic—An anemia induced by the destruction of erythrocytes by chemicals or parasites.
- Hemorrhagic—An anemia induced by loss of erythrocytes either internally or externally.
- Hyperchromic—An anemia characterized by a greater than normal MCH.
- Hypochromic—An anemia characterized by a below normal MCH.
- Iron deficiency—An anemia due to insufficient amounts of serum iron for hemoglobin production. It is characterized by being microcytic and hypochromic.
- Macrocytic—An anemia characterized by higher than normal MCV and the presence of reticulocytes or macrocytes.
- Microcytic—An anemia characterized by a below normal MCV and the presence of microcytic erythrocytes.
- Non-regenerative—An anemia in which there is impaired production of erythrocytes by the bone marrow. It is characterized by the absence or low numbers of reticulocytes in the peripheral blood.
- Normochromic—An anemia characterized by a normal MCH.
- Normocytic—An anemia characterized by a normal MCV.
- Regenerative—An anemia in which there is active production of erythrocytes by the bone marrow. It is characterized by reticulocytosis of the peripheral blood.

Anisocytosis—Variation in size of the erythrocytes.

Anorexia—Loss of appetite.

Antemortem—Before death.

Antibodies—A globulin protein synthesized by

the lymphoid tissue of the body in response to antigenic stimulation.

Antidiuretic Hormone—A hormone produced by the posterior pituitary that increases the permeability of water in the distal tubles and collection ducts of the kidneys and conserves body water.

Antigen—A substance that stimulates the formation of antibodies when it is introduced into the body. Common antigens are bacteria, viruses, fungi, etc.

Anthelmintic—Any drug used for deworming. Synonymous with vermifuge.

Anuria—The absence of urine production.

Aplasia—Cessation of blood-cell formation.

Apochromatic Objective—A lense of higher quality than an achromatic lens and recommended for color photography. Apochromats correct for three colors chromatically and two colors spherically. Special compensating eyepieces must be used with these objectives.

Arrhythmia—Irregularity of cardiac rhythm.

Ascites—Accumulation of fluid within the abdominal cavity.

Autoimmune Hemolytic Anemia—Immunologically mediated anemia characterized by the presence of spherocytes and a positive Coombs test.

Azotemia—The presence of abnormal amounts of non-protein nitrogenous elements in the blood, particularly urea and creatinine.

Band Leukocyte—A leukocyte with a nucleus that is unsegmented and ribbonlike (also called stab or nonfilamented).

Basophil—A granulocytic leukocyte characterized by a large segmented nucleus and basophilic-cytoplasmic granules.

Basophilia—When applied to a cell of the erythrocytic series, this term indicates that the cell shows no trace of characteristic hemoglobin color and the cytoplasm shows a strong affinity for basophilic dyes. With Romanowsky stains, the cytoplasm of these cells stains with various intensities of opaque blue.

Basophilic Stippling—Erythrocytes that have blue-staining, basophilic granules scattered throughout. This indicates lead poisoning in dogs.

Bilirubin—A pigment occuring in bile that is formed from the breakdown of hemoglobin from erythrocytes.

Bolus—A mass administered at one short time.

Bone Marrow—The central portion of long and flat bones and the principle site of blood-cell formation in adult animals.

Bradyarrhythmia—An abnormal rhythm of the heartbeat that occurs when the heart rate is less than 70 beats per minute.

Catabolism—The breakdown of body proteins and fats into more simple compounds. Destructive metabolism.

Catarrhal—Inflammation of mucous membranes with hypersecretion of fluid or mucus.

Cholangitis—Inflammation or infection of the bile ducts of the liver.

Cholestasis—The obstruction (partial or complete) of the flow of bile from the liver into the duodenum.

Chromatic Aberration—A defect caused by the

focusing of different colors of light at different points along the optical axis. High-quality lenses correct these defects by the addition of special types of glass. Poor-quality objectives cause fringes of color around the image.

Chymotrypsinogen—A proenzyme produced by the pancreas and activated to its proteolytic form by trypsin.

Colorimeter—A laboratory instrument that utilizes filters to separate the electromagnetic spectrum of light into a few selected wave lengths and a photocell to detect the amount of light that is transmitted through a laboratory specimen.

Cornified Epithelial Cell—A squamous epithelial cell that has matured to the point of becoming keratinized (degenerate, non-viable).

Crenation—A shrinking of erythrocytes causing sharp spikes and irregular margins, usually caused by improper preservation of blood or smearing technique.

Cushing Disease—An excessive production of glucocorticoid hormones by the adrenal cortex.

Cutaneous Larval Migrans—A mild disease syndrome of humans caused by cutaneous migration of the larvae of Ancylostoma brazilienze.

Cyanosis—A bluish discoloration of the mucous membranes apparent when reduced hemoglobin levels exceed 5 g/dl.

Cystocentesis—The removal of urine from the urinary bladder by perabdominal penetration of the urinary bladder with a syringe and needle or indwelling catheter.

Deciliter—One-hundreth (1/100) of a liter. Equivalent to 100 ml.

Degenerative Left Shift—Increased number of immature leukocytes without a concurrent leukocytosis.

Depolarization—The process of neutralizing polarity and thus contraction.

Dermatomycosis—Infection of the skin with fungal organsims.

Dermatophytosis—Infection of the skin with fungal organisms.

Desquamation—The sloughing off of cells from the tissue.

Diabetes Insipidus—A disease syndrome characterized by insufficient production or utilization of antidiuretic hormone.

Diabetes Mellitus—A persistent hyperglycemia due to either a relative or absolute decrease in insulin production by the beta cells of the pancreas.

Differential Count—A count (in percentage) of the types of leukocytes seen on a stained blood smear or bone marrow.

Dohle Bodies—Small (1 to 2 microns) round or oval, gray-blue bodies in the cytoplasm of the neutrophils thought to be due to incomplete utilization of ribonucleic acid (RNA)during maturation of the cytoplasm.

Dyspnea—Difficult respiration.

ECG 60 Cycle—Sharp movements on a ECG due to electrical interference.

Ecchymotic Hemorrhage—Large areas of superficial hemorrhage.

Eclampsia—Convulsions from a specific cause, usually hypocalcemia.

Ectopic—Located away from normal position.

Edema—Increased amounts of interstitial fluid within the tissues.

Electrocardiogram—A graphic record of the electrical activity of the heart.

Electrocardiology—The study of graphic records made from electrical activity of the heart.

Electrolyte—A solution that can conduct electricity by means of its ions, *i.e.* sodium, chloride, potassium, calcium, etc.

Enteritis—Inflammation of the intestinal tract.

Enterokinase—An enzyme produced by the duodenal mucosa that activates the proenzyme trypsinogen to trypsin, a proteolytic enzyme.

Enzootic—Present in the animal community at all times.

Eosinophil—A granulocytic leukocyte characterized by a segmented nucleus and eosinophilic cytoplasmic granules. In the canine species, the granules are round and of variable size. In the feline species, the granules are rod shaped.

Eosinophilia—An increase in the absolute number of eosinophils in the blood.

Epistaxis—Nosebleed.

Erythrocyte Sedimentation Rate—The rate of sedimentation of erythrocytes when collected in an anticoagulant and placed in a vertical Winthrobe tube for 60 minutes.

Erythroid Hyperplasia—An above normal increase in the number of nucleated erythroid cells over the number of myeloid cells of the bone marrow.

Erythroid Hypoplasia—A decrease number below normal of the nucleated erythroid cells in relation to the myeloid cells of the bone.

Erythropoiesis—The production of erythrocytes.

Erythropoietin—The hormonal substance in the plasma that regulates erythropoiesis by stimulating the bone marrow.

Ethylenediaminetetraacetate—An anticoagulant that prevents coagulation of blood by chelating calcium.

Exudate—An abnormal body fluid that accumulates due to infection or inflammation.

Femtoliter—10^{-15} liters.

French Units—A unit of measure that is frequently used for catheters and endotracheal tubes. One millimeter equals three French units.

Glomerulonephritis—Inflammation or infection of the glomeruli of the kidney.

Glucagon—A hormone produced by the alpha cells of the islets of Langerhans of the pancreas, which elevates blood glucose by stimulating glycogenolysis and gluconeogenesis.

Gluconeogenesis—The production of glucose from non-carbohydrate sources such as amino acids.

Gluten-free—Free of protein from wheat and other grains.

Glycogenolysis—The breakdown of the hepatic and skeletal muscle stores of glycogen.

Granulocyte—A leukocyte that contains specific cytoplasmic granules (neutrophils, eosinophils, basophils) regardless of the stage of differentiation.

Heinz Bodies—An intra-erythrocytic mass of denatured hemoglobin, irregularly shaped, and appearing as refractile granules when slightly out of focus. This latter property is responsible for their also being called *erythrocyte refractile bodies* (ER bodies).

Hemarthrosis—Hemorrhage into the joint capsules.

Hematocrit—The percentage of whole blood that is comprised of erythrocytes.

Hematophagous—Blood sucking.

Hematuria—The presence of blood in the urine.

Hemoglobin—A conjugated protein/iron complex contained within erythrocytes, which serves to transport oxygen and carbon dioxide.

Hemoglobinuria—The presence of hemoglobin in the urine.

Hemolysis—Destruction of the erythrocytes by dissolution or lysis.

Hemophilia A—An inheritable bleeding disorder in which there is a deficiency of Factor VIII.

Hemophilia B—An inheritable bleeding disorder in which there is a deficiency of Factor IX.

Heparin—An anticoagulant that prevents the coagulation of blood by interfering with the conversion of prothrombin to thrombin.

Hepatomegaly—Enlargement of the liver to greater than normal size.

Howell-Jolly Bodies—Small, round, densely staining bodies in the erythrocytes. They are considered to be nuclear remnants.

Hyperchromasia—When applied to cells of the erythrocytic series, this term indicates that the cells have a more intense hemoglobin color. This is not due to increased concentration of hemoglobin, but to increased thickness of the observed cell.

Hyperplasia—Increase in size of an organ or tissue due to increase in the number of cells in the organ or tissue.

Hypertonic—Having an osmotic pressure greater than normal extracellular fluid.

Hypertrophy—Increase in size of an organ or tissue due to increase in the size of the individual cells in the organ or tissue.

Iatrogenic—Induced or caused by the physician.

Icterus—An abnormally high accumulation of bilirubin in the body tissues and blood.

Indices—Calculations of the erythrocyte size, hemoglobin content, and hemoglobin concentration.

Insulin—A hormone produced by the beta cells of the islets of Langerhans of the pancreas that facilitates entry of glucose into body cells.

Intussusception—A telescoping of one part of the intestines into another part of the intestines.

Isothenuria—Urine specific gravity in the glomerular "fixed range" of 1.008 to 1.012, regardless of the osmotic balance of the body.

Isotonic—Osmotically balanced with the normal extracellular fluid.

Jaundice—An abnormally high accumulation of bilirubin in the body tissues and blood.

Jugular Pulse—Pulsations seen in one or both jugular veins due to right heart failure.

Ketoacidosis—The presence of abnormally high amounts of ketones, Beta-hydroxybuteric acid and acetoacetic acid in the body. It usually results from deranged carbohydrate metabolism as seen in diabetes mellitus.

Kussmaul Respiration—Deep respiratory movements seen in conditions of acidosis where the respiratory system is trying to compensate by eliminating excess carbon dioxide gas.

L.E. Cell—A cell seen in systemic lupus erythematosus. It is a phagocyte that has engulfed nuclear protein that is covered with antinuclear antibody.

Leptocyte, Target Cell, or Codocyte—A thin erythrocyte in which the volume is reduced in relationship to the diameter; often characterized by abnormal shape. This shape resembles a target—a central, round, densely pigmented area surrounded by a clear zone that is encircled by a dense ring of pigmented cytoplasm at the periphery of the erythrocyte.

Leukemoid—Resembling leukemia by having a marked leukocytosis or having many immature leukocytes in the peripheral blood, but not due to the same changes in the blood-forming tissues; established that the condition is not true leukemia.

Leukocytosis—An increase in the number of the circulating leukocytes to greater than normal for the species.

Leukopenia—A reduction in the number of circulating leukocytes to less than normal for the species.

Linear Magnification—The product of the magnifications engraved on the objective and eyepiece.

Lipase—A lypolytic enzyme produced in its active form by the pancreas.

Lipemia—The presence of chylomicrons (emulsified fats) in the blood.

Lipolysis—The breakdown of body fat or lysis of dietary absorbed fats.

Lymphangiectasis—Dilatation of the lymphatic vessels.

Lymphoblast—An immature stage of lymphocytes. Their presence in peripheral blood indicates lymphocytic leukemia or lymphosarcoma.

Lymphocyte—An agranulocytic leukocyte characterized by a round nucleus and a basophilic to clear staining cytoplasm.

Lymphocytosis—An increase in the absolute lymphocyte count to a number above normal for the species.

Lymphokine—Cytotoxic substances produced by effector T-lymphocytes.

Lymphopenia—A reduction in the total number of lymphocytes to less than normal for the species.

Macrocyte—An erythrocyte with diameter greater than normal; *i.e.,* reticulocyte.

Malabsorption—Failure of normal absorption of nutrients from the small intestine, in the presence of normal pancreatic enzyme activity.

Maldigestion—Failure of normal digestion or breakdown of nutrients from the small intestines resulting from inadequate pancreatic enzyme activity.

Mean Corpuscular Hemoglobin (MCH)—The hemoglobin content of the average individual erythrocyte expressed in picograms.

Mean Corpuscular Hemoglobin Concentration—The average hemoglobin concentration per deciliter of packed erythrocytes and expressed as a percentage.

Mean Corpuscular Volume (MCV)—The average volume of the individual erythrocyte expressed in femtoliters.

Mean Electrical Activity—The average vector (magnitude and direction) for atrial and ventricular depolarization.

Megakaryocyte—The largest cell of the bone marrow. Cytoplasmic fragments from it form blood platelets or thrombocytes.

Meniscus—The cresent shaped surface of a liquid column.

Metamyelocyte—The first developmental stage of the leukocytic series in which the nucleus begins to indent. It is also known as a juvenile cell and is frequently seen in the peripheral blood of animals with severe infections.

Metarubricyte—The last stage in the erythrocyte development which contains a nucleus; a normoblast.

Methemoglobin—Hemoglobin in which the iron is oxidized to the ferrous state and is unable to transport oxygen or carbon dioxide.

Microcyte—An erythrocyte with diameter less than normal; *i.e.,* spherocyte.

Microliter (μ 1)—One millionth of a liter. Equivalent to a cubic millimeter.

Milliliter—One-thousandths (1/1000) of a liter.

Monocyte—An agranulocytic leukocyte characterized by a large variable-shaped nucleus and a "sky-blue" to light staining cytoplasm that frequently is vacuolated.

Monocytosis—An increase in the absolute monocyte count to a number above normal for the species.

Monomorphism—Denotes the same morphologic character of the principle cell type in the blood, bone marrow, or tissue impression.

Monosaccharides—Simple carbohydrates such as glucose, fructose, etc.

Mycoses—A general term denoting infection with fungal organisms; the infection can be either superficial or systemic.

Myeloblast—The most immature bone marrow stem cell that will develop into one of the leukocytic series.

Myelocyte—The first developmental stage of the leukocytic series in the bone marrow with specific cytoplasmic granules that denotes whether it will develop into a neutrophil, eosinophil, or basophil.

Myeloid Erythroid Ratio—The ratio of the leukocytic (myeloid) cells of the bone marrow to the nucleated red blood cells of the bone marrow.

Myeloid Hyperplasia—An above normal increase in the number of myeloid cells over the nucleated erythroid cells of the bone marrow.

Myeloid Hypoplasia—A decreased number below normal of the myeloid cells in relation to the nucleated erythroid cells of the bone marrow.

Myocarditis—Inflammation of cardiac muscle.

Necropsy—An autopsy.

Necrosis—Death of tissue.

Neoplasia—A new and abnormal growth that is not under normal body control (cancer).

Nephritis—Inflammation or infection of one or both kidneys.

Nephron—The functional unit of the kidney, consisting of a glomerules, proximal convoluted tubule, loop of Henle and distal convoluted tubule.

Neutropenia—A reduction in the total number of neutrophils to less than normal for the species.

Neutrophil—A granulocytic leukocyte characterized by neutral staining cytoplasmic granules and a segmented nucleus.

Neutrophilia—An increase in the total number of neutrophils to more than normal for the species.

Normochromasia—When applied to cells of the erythrocytic series, this term indicates that the cells have their full complement of hemoglobin and no residual basophilic material in the cytoplasm; *i.e.,* they show normal staining characteristics.

Numerical Aperture (NA)—The numbers engraved on the objectives and condensers, which can be used in computing resolution. The NA of the substage condenser must always be greater than that of the objective in use.

Objective—The lens system nearest the object being viewed.

Occult—Hidden, not visible or demonstrable by normal laboratory tests.

Oliguria—A below normal production of urine.

Onychomycosis—Dermatophytosis involving the toenails and nail beds.

Osteodystrophy—Defective bone formation. In renal osteodystrophy there is demineralization of previously normal mineralized bone.

Osteomalacia—A softening of the bones.

Osteosarcoma—Cancer of the bones.

Oxyhemoglobin—Hemoglobin in which the iron is associated with the oxygen molecule in the active transport of oxygen.

Oxylates—Anticoagulants that prevent the coagulation of blood by chelating calcium.

P Mitrale—Left atrial enlargement associated with mitral valve disease.

P Pulmonale—Right atrial enlargement due to right heart or pulmonary disease.

Packed Cell Volume—The percentage of whole blood that is comprised of erythrocytes.

Parenteral—Administration of medication or fluids in a route other than the gastrointestinal tract.

Pelger-Huet Anomaly—A rare hereditary condition associated with a myeloproliferative disorder in which neutrophils lack the usual nuclear segmentation.

Pericarditis—Inflammation of the covering of the heart.

Petechial Hemorrhage—Small "pinpoint" areas of superficial hemorrhage.

Phagocyte—A cell that has the capability of ingesting foreign substances within the body, *i.e.,* neutrophil, macrophage.

Physiologic Leukocytosis—A total leukocyte count above normal without the association of any disease process. It is usually associated with conditions that result in a release of epinephrine with the immediate mobilization of neutrophils that have marginated in small blood vessels and are flushed into the larger blood vessels with the increased blood flow. As a rule, all cell types participate in the increase, but there is a tendency toward a neutrophilia without a shift to the left. Absolute numbers of leukocytes and eosinophils remain normal except in the cat, where a mild lymphocytosis may occur.

Picrogram—10^{-12} grams.

Plan-Achromatic Objective (or Plan-Apochromatic objective)—The prefix plan simply indicates that efforts have been made to create a flat optical field. This is helpful in photomicrography but is an unnecessary expense in a clinical instrument.

Plasma—The non-cellular portion of anticoagulated blood.

Poikilocyte—An erythrocyte with an abnormal shape; not to be confused with distortion resulting from crenation.

Polyarthritis—Inflammation of more than one of the synovial joints of the body.

Polychromasia—Variation in color among erythrocytes resulting from the admixture of normal staining erythrocytes with the more basophilic reticulocytes.

Polycythemia—An increased number of erythrocytes per microliter of blood.

Polydipsia—An above normal daily consumption of water (> than 50ml/lb/day for dogs).

Polymyositis—Inflammation of the muscles of the body.

Polyphagia—An above normal increase in appetite and food consumption.

Polypnea—Panting or abnormally rapid respiration.

Polyuria—An above normal daily production of urine (> than 25ml/lb/day for dogs).

Post-morten—After death. Also refers to an autopsy or necropsy.

Postprandial—After eating a meal.

Prepatent Period—The period of time from infection by a parasite until it matures and passes ova into the feces or sputum.

Procarboxypeptidases—Proenzymes produced by the pancreas and activated to their proteolytic form by trypsin.

Progranulocyte—A developmental stage of leukocytes characterized by a large round nucleus and azure cytoplasmic granules. This cell can develop into a neutrophilic, eosinophilic, or basophilic myelocyte.

Prorubricyte—Second nucleated stage in the development of the erythrocyte.

Proteinuria—The presence of protein in the urine.

Pruritus—An itching sensation.

Pyelonephritis—Inflammation or infection of the renal pelvis and collecting ducts.

Pyrexia—Abnormally high body temperature. A fever.

Reduced Hemoglobin—Hemoglobin in which the iron is unassociated with the oxygen molecule and the heme component is reversibly combined with carbon dioxide.

Refractometer—A laboratory instrument that measures the amount of light refraction through a laboratory specimen.

Regenerative Left Shift—Increased numbers of immature leukocytes in the presence of a leukocytosis.

Repolarization—The process of re-establishing polarity in cardiac cells.

Resolution—The ability of a lens to reveal fine detail without blurring.

Reticulocyte—Any non-nucleated erythrocyte containing enough RNA that, when it is supravitally stained with new methylene blue or brilliant cresyl blue, it will have discernible granules or a diffuse network of fibrils.

Rouleau formation—The arrangement of erythrocytes in a roll or column resembling a stack of coins.

Rubriblast—First nucleated stage in the development of the erythrocyte.

Rubricyte—The nucleated stages of the erythrocyte in which the hemoglobin is formed.

Sedimentation Rate—The rate at which erythrocytes fall in their own plasma in a given length of time.

Serum—The non-cellular portion of clotted blood.

Shift to the Left—An increase in the immature forms of the granulocytic leukocytes in the blood.

Shift to the Right—An increase in the percent of older leukocytes (hypersegmentation) in the blood.

Simple Substage Condenser (ABBE)—A condenser that has no correction for chromatic or spherical aberrations. It is satisfactory for most visual work if the NA exceeds that of the objective being used. It should not be used with planachromatic or epochromatic objectives.

Sinus Rhythm—A "p" wave for every QRS complex and a QRS comples for every "p" wave.

Smudge Cell—A ruptured leukocyte.

Specific Gravity—The weight of a liquid compared with that of distilled water.

Spectrophotometer—A laboratory instrument that uses prisms to separate the different wave lengths of light and a photocell to detect the amount of light that is transmitted through a laboratory specimen.

Spherical Aberration—A defect in the capability of a lens to concentrate light at a central point, which results in a blurred image.

Spherocyte—A spheroid erythrocyte of decreased diameter in relationship to its volume and having the microscopic appearance of a hyperchromatic microcyte.

Splenomegaly—Enlargement of the spleen to greater than normal size.

Split Plate—Combinations of different materials capable of helping in differentiation of microbes.

Sputum—Salivary secretions mixed with matter ejected from the lungs, bronchi, and trachea.

Stab Cell—The band form of a granulocyte.

Steatorrhea—Undigested fat particles in the stool in amounts greater than normal.

Stomatocyte—Erythrocytes with a shape deformity in which there is a linear rather than a central area of pallor.

Subcutis—The tissue immediately below the epidermis and dermis

Supraventricular—Pertaining to abnormalities relating to the atria.

Syncope—Fainting.

Syncytium—A merging of cells toward a single functional goal.

Tachyarrhythmia—An abnormal rhythm of the heartbeat that occurs when the heart rate is greater than 160 beats per minute.

Telogen—The resting phase of a hair follicle.

Thrombasthenin—A protein released by thrombocytes that aids in clot retraction.

Thrombocytopathy—Defective thrombocyte function but normal thrombocyte counts in the peripheral blood.

Thrombocytopenia—A decrease in number of thrombocytes (platelets) below the normal for the species.

Toxic neutrophil—A neutrophil characterized by toxic granules, basophilia of the cytoplasm, vacuoles, or condensation of nuclear chromatin.

Transudate—A normal body fluid that accumulates due to altered osmotic pressures.

Trypsinogen—The proenzyme form of the proteolytic enzyme trypsin.

Uremia—The presence of abnormal amounts of urea in the blood.

Urobilin—A brown pigment formed by oxidation of urobilinogen. This imparts the normal color to feces.

Urobilinogen—A colorless compound formed in the intestines by the reduction of bilurbin.

Uropathy—A disease or disorder of the urinary tract.

Vasoconstriction—Constriction of the small blood vessels.

Vasodilation—Dilatation of the small blood vessels.

Vasopressor—Medications used to increase peripheral blood pressure.

Vector—Magnitude and force of electrical activity.

Venodilation—Dilation of the small venules.

Ventricular—Pertaining to abnormalities relating to the ventricles.

Visceral Larval Migrans—A mild disease syndrome of humans caused by deep migration of the larvae of Toxocara canis.

Whipples Triad—A series of signs consisting of neurologic disturbances, fasting blood glucose $<$ 40 mg/dl and cessation of neurologic signs upon administration of glucose or feeding. Seen in hypoglycemia syndromes.

Wood Light—An ultraviolet light of 3600 Angstrom unit wavelength that is filtered through nickel oxide. Used to demonstrate the presence or absence of fluoresence in superficial fungal infections.

INDEX

A

B

* denotes GLOSSARY

C

D

E

F

* denotes GLOSSARY

G

H

I

J

K

L

M

* denotes GLOSSARY

N

O

P

Q

R

S

* denotes GLOSSARY

T

U

V

W

NOTES